D1174097

Operating on the Mind

OPERATING
ON
THE MIND

The
Psychosurgery Conflict

EDITED BY

WILLARD M. GAYLIN, JOEL S. MEISTER,

AND ROBERT C. NEVILLE

Basic Books, Inc., Publishers   *New York*

This book was prepared with the support of the National Science Foundation Grant No. GI34276X1. However, any opinions, findings, conclusions, or recommendations expressed herein are those of the authors and do not necessarily reflect the views of the National Science Foundation.

Library
I.U.P.
Indiana, Pa.

174.2 Op2e
c.1

Library of Congress Cataloging in Publication Data
Main entry under title:

Operating on the mind.

Includes bibliographies and index.
1. Psychiatric ethics. 2. Psychosurgery.
I. Gaylin, Willard M. II. Meister, Joel S. III. Neville,
Robert C. [DNLM: 1. Psychosurgery. 2. Ethics,
Medical. WL370 061]
RC455.2.P77064   174'.2   74-79276
ISBN 0-465-05288-6

© 1975 by the Institute of Society, Ethics
and the Life Sciences
Printed in the United States of America
Designed by Vincent Torre
75 76 77 78 79   10 9 8 7 6 5 4 3 2 1

CONTENTS

Preface   vi

1 / The Problem of Psychosurgery   3
  WILLARD M. GAYLIN, M.D.

2 / Psychosurgery and Brain Stimulation in
    Historical Perspective   24
    HERBERT G. VAUGHAN, JR., M.D.

3 / Kaimowitz v. Department of Mental
    Health: The Detroit Psychosurgery Case   73
    RONALD S. GASS

4 / Zalmoxis or The Morals of ESB and
    Psychosurgery   87
    ROBERT C. NEVILLE, Ph.D.

5 / Regulating Psychosurgery: Issues of
    Public Policy and Law   117
    HAROLD EDGAR, LL.D.

6 / The Need for Policy   169
    JOEL S. MEISTER, Ph.D.

Appendix   185
Index   210

PREFACE

THE CENTRAL PROBLEM of this book is the worthiness of psychosurgery as a therapeutic modality. It has been clear to us from the beginning that the "worthiness of psychosurgery" is not merely a question of medical cost-benefit analysis. Rather, there are many serious questions, such as how these techniques affect the social definition of mental illness in comparison to the influence of psychoanalytic thinking, or whether these techniques may lend themselves to social abuse in the guise of therapy. In attempting to assess psychosurgery, this book addresses questions related to the state of the art, philosophical presuppositions, social and legal control, and policy formulation.

The studies presented here are the results of a genuinely cooperative effort by the Behavior Control Research Group of the Institute of Society, Ethics and the Life Sciences. The issues and drafts have been discussed so much that we find ourselves quoting each other and wondering who was the original author of some phrase or point. Nevertheless, joint work does not entail agreement, only an understanding of the grounds of disagreement. The chapters here are signed by the individuals taking final responsibility for them. This book is not the "conclusions" of the Research Group, but the diverse results of intensive study of a central problem by investigators from different fields. It should be noted that the authors represent psychiatry, neurology, investigative journalism, philosophy, law, and sociology.

In the end, psychosurgery and other forms of physical manipulation of the brain raise social, political, and economic questions as well as scientific ones. These issues are sorted out both historically and systematically by Willard M. Gaylin in the introductory chapter. Dr. Gaylin is Professor of Psychiatry at

Columbia College of Physicians and Surgeons and the President of the Institute of Society, Ethics and the Life Sciences.

The various social issues surrounding our topic should not obscure the fact that psychosurgery is a medical procedure, and part of the relevant controversy concerns just *how scientific* it is, *whether we know* how scientific it is, and *what its effects are* relative to various conditions and alternate therapies. These scientific issues are addressed by Herbert G. Vaughan, Jr., in Chapter 2.

Dr. Vaughan is Professor of Neurology at Albert Einstein College of Medicine and a founding Fellow of the Institute of Society, Ethics and the Life Sciences. From the standpoint of a clinical investigator, he describes both the history and present state of the art of psychosurgery and electrical stimulation of the brain, such as it can be known, and considers as well some of the effects on scientific medicine of the social issues raised by these technologies.

As chance would have it, during the winter of 1972-1973 a specific case involving both psychosurgery and electrical brain stimulation was brought to public attention and became a cause célèbre. A Detroit neurologist proposed to implant electrodes in the brain of a person institutionalized as a criminal sexual psychopath, for the purpose of diagnostic stimulation to see whether the person would be a candidate for psychosurgery to cure his pathology. This proposal was part of a larger research plan to compare the effectiveness of psychosurgical procedures to a drug producing the effects of castration in controlling criminal sexuality.

The case not only raised the scientific issues of how to define and diagnose the pathological condition, and whether the surgery would work, but it also raised the social questions of therapy in a closed institution; of informed consent; and of the use of prisoners for experimentation. The case came to court and resulted in a striking judicial decision. The story of this case is told in Chapter 3 by Ronald S. Gass, a recent graduate of Duke University and a student intern at the Institute.

The use of psychosurgery strikes at the heart of our basic moral conceptions, and these conceptions must be examined before legal and policy issues can be faced rationally. The moral questions regarding these techniques divide into those raised by their use, or abuse, for nontherapeutic purposes such as the protection of society. Underlying both of these kinds of issues, however, is the deeper problem of the relation between an alteration of a person's brain and the alteration of his person: is the soul under attack? These questions are sorted out and discussed in Chapter 4 by Robert Neville, Professor of Philosophy at the State University of New York at Purchase.

In light of all the problems—social and scientific—occasioned by psychosurgery, what protections do potential patients and society have beyond the obvious ones of self-regulation of the medical community and the patient's power of noncooperation? The ultimate protection is in the law. But should these techniques be regulated by statute? Is there appropriate precedent in case law? Should there be legally authoritative regulative bodies or peer review systems? These issues are addressed in Chapter 5 by Harold Edgar, Professor of Law at Columbia University School of Law and a Fellow of the Institute.

After all the technical, historical, moral, and legal issues have been discussed, what should be done? Is there a need for anything to be done, or will the natural social forces operative in the medical and legal communities take care of things? What things need taking care of? Who should be concerned about the use of psychosurgery? What kinds of regulations would be appropriate and for what groups? Joel S. Meister discusses these and other problems of policy in Chapter 6. As it turns out, the thorniest problem is defining the scope of psychosurgery in the first place, a problem implicit throughout this book. Dr. Meister is the Associate for Behavioral Sciences at the Institute and Staff Director of the Behavior Control Research Group.

Our final chapter ought to be the "bottom line" where the answers are given. But the real result of our research has been to see where the problems are. We are not policy makers, but we do hope that this book will clarify many of the issues in the psychosurgery conflict, issues which must be resolved eventually by those who do make policy.

Operating on the Mind

WILLARD M. GAYLIN, M.D.

1 / The Problem of Psychosurgery

SOME FORMS of behavior control have existed throughout human history. Man is an obligate social animal; people are as essential to his survival as oxygen. Compelled by his biological structure to spend a larger proportion of his lifespan in a state of dependency than any other animal, his very survival as an individual and a species requires a social structure. As soon as it is necessary for people to live together in groups, even if the group is the minimum one of the family, there will exist the need for codes of behavior defining what is permissible and what is not.

The systems of control now used are multiple and overlapping. They include volitional controls exercised by the individual to satisfy certain internalized standards, obligatory external controls such as the laws of the society with their built-in rewards and punishments, and an ambiguous and pervasive set of social controls (e.g., peer pressure) which are external, operate without the mandate of law, but nonetheless often have the impelling force of law. Even the internal controls were in great part originally externally produced, since the defined values of the society determine the nature of the ideals and aspirations programmed into the individual. Culture is man's creator as surely as it is his creation. The capacity for man's control of man provides great opportunity for improving the human condition, but has led to ethical considerations of its permissibility, and protective measures against its abuse. In all of this there is nothing new. What is new is the growing magnitude of the problem.

As is true of all aspects of the biological revolution, it is the success of science that confounds us. The urgency of the problem in behavior control results from our recent advances in knowledge and technology. Everywhere, it is the success of science and medicine that confronts old issues of man's nature and autonomy.

Knowledge of what motivates man. The increased knowledge of depth psychology has permitted the evaluation of human motivation and development at a level of understanding previously possible only in studies of physiological behavior.

Techniques to apply the knowledge. The sophisticated knowledge of how to control human behavior by the manipulation of emotions and the induction of reward and punishment programs has progressed rapidly in the last 50 years. It has been augmented by the use of drugs of a progressively more specialized nature. This can now be supplemented by the potential for direct electrical stimulation of the brain, with its promise of remote control electronic devices.

Psychological readiness to accept new forms of behavior control. Invariably when the problem of behavior control is anticipated, it is visualized in science fiction terms: some dictatorial authority operating on the brains of individuals to create human automatons. In reality, however, it will not evolve this way. The great innovations in social behavior are traditionally voluntary and, good or bad, are usually first introduced in the *name* of good. Psychosurgery, our current example, was initiated originally not to create populations of robots but to free patients from the chains of schizophrenia. As long as each phenomenon is considered on an ad hoc basis, its full implications will never be faced; each specific instance will appear as a desirable step, not as a possible threat. Introduced in the name of health and welfare, these advances will for the most part be invited, even demanded. Contributing to this rapid evolution will be the tendency for technology always to demand fulfillment of that which is possible. More important, the philosophy of the time will encourage it.

With the dissipation of traditional religious influences, the design of God has been replaced by the purposes of man—and health, survival, pleasure, and performance of the individual become central considerations.

Growth of mass delivery methods. Drugs, for instance, are administered not only through ad hoc doctor-patient relationships but also through the policies of school systems, e.g., vaccinations for polio and sedative drugs in certain cases.

Social critics have long called attention to the potential exploitation of the mass media for indoctrination. The example is set by the increasing surreptitious use, in advertising, of psychological fears and inducements to create false need. Even sexual mores, for example, are not now exclusively determined by local custom, but also by the influence, communicated through mass media, of a smaller group of experts or "taste makers."

Furthermore, *access* to the means and facilities for influencing behavior has come to be restricted to a smaller percentage of the population as those means have become progressively more effective in influencing a larger and larger percentage of the society.

Specific dangers are often self-evident. Some dangers, however, are so abstract and incremental as to become apparent only when near the brink. This is particularly true when the common problems arise in isolated and disparate areas. Think, for example, of the field of ecology. For years agronomists had been concerned with soil erosion, marine biologists with the contamination of rivers and streams, urbanologists with the destruction of the central city, respiratory physiologists with contaminants in the air, and geologists with the exhaustion of energy resources. These men, dealing in different technologies and often with different languages, were not readily aware of the common features of the environmental problem. As a result they were unprepared to alert the public to the common danger. Only when the sum total began to be put together, and the concept emerged that the earth itself was a limited and precious resource which we were wantonly destroying, did the totality of the threat begin to be taken seriously—thus was born the "ecology movement."

The time has come for a comparable recognition in the field of behavior control. Psychiatrists, brain physiologists, sociologists, psychologists, political scientists, lawyers, pharmacologists, and educators, among others, have been concerned in their separate ways and in their separate fields about the growing capacity to control behavior, its potential mass utilization, and the capacity for misuse inherent in such potential. Yet so far they have lacked a common framework of questions with which they might focus their concerns and exchange their findings. So far the wider public has lacked the clarifying concepts which might alert it to the need for exploring certain possibilities and anticipating certain dangers. What should be seen as a common problem is handled in bits and pieces. To employ a recent catch phrase, it is necessary to "get it together."

To this end the Institute of Society, Ethics and the Life Sciences established a Behavior Control Research Program which set as its goals: (1) development of an adequate perspective or theory for conceptualizing human behavior relative to the methods and technologies for controlling it; (2) assessment of the benefits and liabilities of various behavior controls relative to the values of our society; and (3) discovering ways of incorporating our values about behavior control into the institutions and mores of our society. Six specific spheres were to be explored. They were: (1) physical manipulation of the brain; (2) chemical manipulation of the brain; (3) psychological control; (4) control through total institutions; (5) control through media; and (6) control through educational institutions.

It is to the first of these, and specifically to psychosurgery (more than electrode implantation), that this book is addressed. Psychosurgery itself is probably, at this point, less important in terms of either its potential uses or potential abuses than most other procedures capable of manipulating or modifying behavior. Nonetheless, because of the narrowness of its current procedures, the relatively limited number of variables, and the dramatic nature of its technique, it serves as a focusing lens to sharpen the image of long-existing problems which have been neglected in other more traditional areas. These areas of concern include two broad and diverse fields: First, psychosurgery is a prototype, at its most extreme, of all behavior modification, and suggests all the problems inherent in the other forms of behavior control and, indeed, in some forms of education and rehabilitation. Further, it also serves to focus problems existing in other forms of surgery, and while this is not the primary purpose of our discussion here, the policy implications can be clearly seen to be readily extendable beyond psychosurgery into neurosurgery and, beyond that, into the general control of all surgical procedures. Chapter 5 includes an extensive discussion of this issue. Psychosurgery thus becomes an ideal excuse, and mechanism, to reexamine the surgical contract, particularly in comparison with relative attitudes toward drugs and other forms of therapy.

But psychosurgery demands attention in its own right. Any procedure which has the potential for such immediate, direct, and dramatic alteration of both behavior and personality warrants more careful attention than has been given in the past. While psychosurgery may be similar to other forms of behavior modification, the *immediacy* of its effect and the totality of control possible suggest a coercive potential beyond that inherent in the more gradual procedures.

At this point it might be well to describe and define what we are talking about—what *is* psychosurgery? Here we are already in difficulty. As will be elaborated in later chapters, the definition of psychosurgery has varied from one individual surgeon to another, and enormous complications have arisen in the discourse simply because of the failure to define the term clearly. It is not an easy term to define. Initially, it may be thought of as surgical destruction of certain portions of the brain for purposes of treating psychiatric conditions. The problems of definition are addressed by Harold Edgar in his analysis of legal issues (Chapter 5) and by Joel Meister in his discussion of policy issues (Chapter 6). The detailed elaboration of the nature of current surgical procedures available, the anticipated positive modifications possible with each procedure, and the negative side effects of the procedures are discussed by Dr. Herbert Vaughan (Chapter 2).

Technically, the procedures are not considered difficult. The original psychosurgery which attracted the most attention was the prefrontal lobotomy done in the 1930s and 1940s. It was essentially a crude cutting of tracks of the frontal lobe, a gross procedure done usually without direct observation but by estimation from external measurements of the skull. The procedure was simple enough. Prefrontal lobotomy is done under a local anesthetic and can be performed as an office procedure, particularly when the probe is introduced into the orbit above the eyeball where the skull is particularly thin. Dr. Walter Freeman,[2] the pioneer who had done thousands of these procedures, was not even a surgeon, but a professor of neurology at George Washington University Medical School.

Modern procedures are much more elaborate, much more localized, and in that sense much less destructive. They interrupt neural pathways at various levels of the limbic system, a poorly understood, extensive system of nuclear centers and connecting tracks that is known to mediate much of man's emotional life. This is now done either through opening the skull for direct observation, or with complicated stereotactic devices that permit a three-dimensional view, via x-rays, of the inserted instruments.[4] Part of the confusion in some of the more rhetorical attacks on psychosurgery is that it has not always been made clear that the recommended surgery is not the prefrontal lobotomy—that crude instrument of the previous day. It should be remembered, however, in defense of those pioneering surgeons, that when the prefrontal lobotomy was first introduced it was used in a limited number of extremely deteriorated backward patients for whom nothing else seemed to avail.

Unfortunately for these patients, the first of the major tranquilizers soon emerged which proved capable of handling many of the same patients in less dramatic fashion. Had the tranquilizers not been developed it is conceivable that—restricted to this small segment of the psychiatric population—even those crude, simple prefrontal lobotomies might be defensible today. Of course, drugs *were* developed, and that in itself is a significant and cogent indictment against any more drastic procedure. Medical knowledge is in a constant state of expansion—and the promise of the future must place some limits on procedures of the present. More important, while the operation might have had some validity as a treatment of last resort in a desperately deteriorated population, it was not so limited. The urgent hope for the dramatic and the magical in patients; the seductiveness of the

8

facile and quick procedure for the psychiatrist; the exploitation of the easy and the profitable by the least competent therapist led, as it did in shock treatment, to a sickening abuse of this procedure. While it may not be fair to judge a scientific procedure by the abuses to which it *might* lead, it seems reasonable to judge it on the basis of abuses to which it is *likely* to lead.

Certain crucial statistical facts about any new procedures would seem essential before making judgments as to worth. What psychological conditions actually exist for which these procedures might be used, and what is the incidence of these conditions? What are the exact sequelae of each procedure, the potential dangers, the limit of risks? We do not even know how many have been performed. The estimates run from 200 to 1,000.[1,7] There is no organized follow-up except at the discretion of individual surgeons. Which surgeons are performing what operation? Where? And for what purposes? Again, we do not know, since there is no central registry for surgical procedures of any sort.

How can adequate studies be conducted of the effectiveness of psychosurgical procedures when control groups are virtually impossible to define, given the individual quality of so much mental illness? How can even anecdotal evidence be assessed when negative results are not systematically reported? How can reasonable evaluations be made of persons while still in a restrictive institutional setting, when the concern is to discover how they would behave outside the institutions?

Obviously some of these questions can be directed to all forms of psychotherapy, but they tend to be magnified by the irreversible nature of a procedure like psychosurgery, making a mistake all the more poignant. Certainly some tighter procedural methods must be established before we can even begin to consider the still profound problems that will inevitably remain.

From its inception in 1936, psychosurgery has been a controversial medical therapy. The initial question of its effectiveness and dangers immediately became intertwined with second-order questions of how one determines whether it has been effective, and how one measures side effects. Traditionally, such discussions have been exclusively the concern of the medical profession. Disagreements about the protocol, efficacy, or ethics of any given technique may have produced controversy among surgeons, but the public has rarely been involved. By the early 1970s the controversy had taken on a political and social quality, with charges that psychosurgery might be used to induce docility in mental patients, political demonstrators, and whole classes of people who are particularly powerless to resist. Dr. Peter Breggin, a practicing psychiatrist in Washington, D.C., was primarily responsible for turning psychosurgery from a clinical into a political issue. Dr. Breggin's 25,000 word denunciation of psychosurgery was inserted in the *Congressional Record* by Representative Cornelius Gallagher in 1971.[1] In that document he condemned a procedure that he considered experimental, with few reports of results or serious side effects. Arguing for a moratorium on psychosurgery, he criticized any surgery that "blunts" the highest part of man, viewing such psychosurgery as a potential method of social control against young people, women, and blacks.

Concern over the issue by lawmakers resulted in the introduction of two bills in Congress. A House bill flatly prohibiting psychosurgery in most hospitals was sponsored by Representative Louis Stokes (D-Ohio) and 18 other congressmen. Anyone who violated the ban would be fined up to $10,000. In addition, anyone performing psychosurgery would be ineligible for grants, contracts, loans, or guarantees made by the government for five years after date of the violation.

Senate Joint Resolution 86, calling for a two-year moratorium on federal aid for projects involving psychosurgery, was introduced by Senator J. Glenn Beall (D-Md.). It called for an evaluation by the Secretary of Health, Education, and Welfare of psychosurgical procedures done in the past five years, and a report to Congress on "the circumstances (if any) in which the performance of psychosurgery is appropriate."

The California legislature had at this same time become involved in the psychosurgery controversy. The Neuropsychiatric Institute at the University of California at Los Angeles was proposing a center for the study and reduction of violence. According to Louis Jolyon West, chairman of the UCLA Department of Psychiatry, the center was designed to study the social and psychological as well as the biological factors involved in violence. Although Dr. West has disassociated psychosurgery from the center, public reaction to psychosurgery was partly responsible for the magnitude of the organized opposition to the center. As a result, the chairman of the California State Senate Health and Welfare Committee asked for a withholding of the $750,000 for the center pending investigation of certain proposed research projects.

Thus the limelight of publicity brought out the political overtones and implications of psychosurgery. Congressional hearings, court cases, and popular magazine articles provided critics of psychosurgery forums for presenting their view. Whether the result will be long overdue regulation of a risky experimental procedure or unjustified suppression of a legitimate therapeutic technique depends on one's own (by now) emotional reaction to psychosurgery. At the very least, however, problems of psychosurgery must be understood not merely according to a model of medical therapy, but according to a social model that registers its nontherapeutic modifications as well.

Here, then, the ethical basis of the problem becomes immediately apparent. To talk about behavior control is to introduce at once considerations of values and ethics. Where behavior must be controlled for social living, the degree and direction of control will always be shaped and balanced by a view of man. Different cultures value different things, and those values are reflected explicitly in their laws and implicitly in their social directives. Differing economic and political systems will value the freedom of the individual as opposed to the common good in varying degrees. The priority placed on the welfare of the individual versus the welfare of the state; survival of the individual versus the pleasure of the individual; the freedom of the individual versus the security of the state; all of these shifting values will influence our attitudes toward psychosurgery. As we begin to sort some of these problems it becomes obvious that it is not just that ethical issues influence medical decisions, but rather that the two are often inseparable. Dr. Robert Veatch has stated,[8] perhaps rightly, that there are no medical decisions which do *not* include value judgments and moral stands.

The number and forms of the dilemmas are almost limitless. To give some coherence to the value problems posed by psychosurgery, a classification of major issues is presented.

The Problem of Consent

It is an accepted practice in medicine that no procedure be done on an individual without his informed consent. Indeed, to do so constitutes assault and battery and is punishable by law. There are certain rights the law currently vests in the individual over his life, his body, and his future. His consent implies that he has executed his best judgment, and his agreement to the procedure is voluntary. The "informed" modifier is considered crucial, particularly in such issues as health, to insure that the individual's judgment is not based on ignorance or deception.

Informed consent is a labyrinth of confusion entered here only reluctantly. It demands volumes of attention, not casual paragraphs. It is of concern in every medical procedure. What does informed mean? How informed? In what language? How much information? Is total information possible? Is it understandable? Would too much information be intimidating? How can we measure the effect of delivering the information or the amount of it perceived? And then there is the consent. Can it be free with a frightened patient? Can it ever be free? Isn't there always a coercive aspect inherent in the authoritarian position of the physician? Can the physician present a bias-free case? Can the helpless patient exercise judgment independent of his doctor? This does not even begin to suggest the extent of this problem.

If the problem is a serious one in general medicine, it is compounded when one thinks of the special conditions of psychosurgery. It is one thing to recognize the difficulties of consent when one is dealing with a whole, intelligent human being who is concerned about a damaged liver, but where psychosurgery is considered, the consenting organ *is* the damaged organ. But to what extent is it damaged, and should this damage impede our acceptance of informed consent?

If the damage is severe enough we revert to a procedure accepted by law—that of proxy consent. Proxy consent is the method used for those people not considered responsible enough to execute judgment of a serious nature about their future. The proxy is invested in their next of kin. The basic assumption is that there is a congruence of interests and identity, shaped by love, between the proxy and the patient. The ideal model is probably a small baby as the patient with its mother as its proxy. Obviously, even with this ideal model there are difficulties. For example, the law grants the competent adult the privilege of death if he so chooses. Even in our ideal case we would be reluctant to grant this permission to a proxy. As we move away from the ideal model, even less drastic procedures force a distinction between proxy and patient. Do we really want to give a mother proxy rights over a seventeen-year-old in all conditions? A seventeen-year-old who is pregnant and wants an abortion? A seventeen-year-old who wishes to use birth control technologies?

When we come to the full adult the problems are even further compounded. If it is a severely crippled, emotionally incompetent adult, it may well be that we can approximate the mother-infant relationship, but most severely ill mental patients are not at all like infants, and while the intellectual insufficiencies may seem as great, the emotional components of the "self" are often vastly different. Mental illness is a fragmented, irrational combination of intact and destroyed faculties. The distinction between a child and an incompetent adult has been grossly neglected by both medicine and law. It is essential that these distinctions be considered in procedures of psychosurgery, where we must balance emotional gains versus emotional prices for which there are few objective measurements, but mainly subjective evaluations.

The Distinction Between Experimental and Therapeutic

The problem of proxy leads directly to the confusion between therapeutic and experimental procedures. The word "experimental" is in itself confusing since it is used in two distinctly different

13

ways. Human subjects can be used for experimental purposes where the research, while humanitarian in intent, serves no specific therapeutic purpose for them—for example, volunteers who test the immunity of vaccines. "Experimental" can also be distinguished from "therapeutic" in the manner used for drugs, where it means that its therapeutic value (or its harmful side effects) have not been proved out. In the preceding discussion of consent it is obvious that wherever we were to draw the line on proxy consent, one significant factor would be whether the procedure were therapeutic or experimental in either sense of the word. We are obviously more likely to grant permission to do a procedure without the consent of the patient, i.e., by proxy consent, if that procedure is essentially aimed at his own good. Even in the model of the infant and the adult, where decisions are typically vested in the parent, many feel that the proxy consent should be outlawed for experimental procedures which do not serve the individual directly. It is one thing to offer oneself in the service of humanity; it is a less generous gesture to offer someone else to that end.

But the clear separation between standards of experimental and therapeutic which have been maintained in the drug example are unbelievably muddled in surgery. Consider the recent discussions concerning surgery for revascularization of the heart. This is a difficult procedure used generally in patients crippled with severe angina. It is done with the hope that it may defer future infarctions. When originally conceived, this operation carried a high mortality rate. It had a 100 percent morbidity rate, since that is the nature of surgery. It was seen by one and all—patients, surgeons, referring physicians—as an experimental procedure. However, certain surgical teams perfected the technique to a point at which the mortality rate in this very sick group was reduced to around 10 percent. With such dramatic improvement, the attitude of referring physicians changed so that in some localities it became viewed as a standard therapeutic option. Compare now how different our attitude would be if we were discussing a drug therapy. If it were suggested that a drug is available which would relieve the symptoms of angina, with some promise, but no evidence, that it might deter future infarctions, would anyone be reassured by the fact that it caused 100 percent morbidity and *only* 10 percent mortality? Would the drug even be marketable?

The operative procedure is not considered experimental because our whole bias toward surgery is different from what it is toward drugs, and for very obvious reasons. Prior to the modern era a control mechanism over surgery analagous to that over drugs would have been unnecessary and foolish. Surgery was a therapy of last resort—often more dreaded than the disease to which it was directed. If the pain and the shock of the operation did not kill you, the postoperative sepsis was likely to. The terror of the patient was sufficient control over the procedure. Now, with the advent of sophisticated anesthesia, antisepsis, and antibiotics, serious surgical interventions, such as prefrontal lobotomy, can be an office procedure. Here again the limited area of psychosurgery may point to deficiencies in our control over the much broader and, in that sense, more significant area of general surgery.

If proper attention had been paid to distinctions between experimental and therapeutic, much of the often confused and more esoteric debate about psychosurgery would not have been necessary, but would have been resolved at this first-line consideration. Nor would it be necessary to advocate, as have some legislators, the "outlawing" of psychosurgery (particularly since what should be outlawed is never adequately defined, and usually includes procedures that are generally agreed to be humanitarian). Careful guidelines drawing, among other things, the distinction between the experimental and therapeutic would probably outlaw the majority, if not all, of the psychosurgery that has caused so much recent debate.

The Organic Versus Nonorganic Problem

Nowhere has the medical issue been joined with the social, ethical, and political issues more dramatically than in the ongoing debate over the work of Drs. Ervin, Mark, and Sweet* on the relationship

*NIMH awarded $500,000 to the Neuro-Research Foundation in Boston, Mass., 1971-1973, to study and control violent behavior that results from brain dysfunction.

of violence to temporal lobe epilepsy.[4] In this work they associate the violent behavior of the temporal lobe epileptic to the convulsive seizure of the frontal lobe epileptic, and state that just as surgical destruction of areas of the frontal lobe may be indicated to control those seizures, surgical destruction of temporal lobe centers may be indicated to control violence. As a safeguard against accusations that the surgery may be used as a means of social control rather than medical therapy (to be discussed later), Dr. Mark, in particular, had been insistent that the surgery not be done unless there is an established organic focus.

This is a particularly interesting and confusing stipulation, for the distinctions between organic and nonorganic are not the architectural, gross ones of the nineteenth century, nor are they simply the anatomical ones which are most readily available to a surgeon. They may rather be located in a chemical system that is not yet identified as structurally "organic" yet is obviously as organic as a gross tissue change.

Even if we follow the simpler models of general surgery, we see that the demand of Breggin[1] and others that psychosurgery be limited to the extirpation of abnormal tissue carries illogicalities with it. First, all surgery destroys healthy tissue. One must tie off normal blood vessels, cut through normal skin, and separate connective tissue before one gets to internal areas. The model that seems the most acceptable to critics of psychosurgery is the removal of a space-occupying lesion. Here indeed is a mass that is abnormal in form and function; its presence interferes with normal function and its removal permits the normal body mechanisms to be maintained. An example would be the removal of a benign brain tumor when expanding pressure causes damage to normal tissue. But there are other quite different models of legitimate surgery. For example, in a paralysis or weakness of an eye muscle which cannot be corrected, one way to improve vision is to shorten the opposing and healthy eye muscle. Or an individual with paralysis of extensor muscles of the arm with painful contractures may require altering the normal flexor muscles of the arm. The arm is still as useless, but the pain and deformity are relieved. An individual with peptic ulcer in his duodenum may have his healthy stomach removed because the functions of the stomach in secreting hydrochloric acid (due to conditions unknown but often psychologically aggravated) encourage ulceration of the duodenal wall. In certain blood dyscrasias, without understanding the exact mechanism, but on a purely pragmatic basis, the removal of a seemingly healthy and normal spleen will cause remission of the problem.

Similarly, in creative and corrective surgery, a shoulder may be functionally repaired by grossly distorting the normal architecture of its musculature; i.e., when an essential muscle has been destroyed, another muscle, normally serving an entirely different but less important function, may be reinserted, thus allowing the patient gradually and artificially to learn to control that muscle to perform the more needed function.

Similarly, healthy skin will be removed from the buttocks, where it is less essential, and grafted to an area of a deforming scar on the face. The examples are almost endless. The purpose of all of these examples is to demonstrate that it is the *functioning* of the individual that concerns us, and that we do not treat some theoretical organic integrity. So is it true with epilepsy—we are not treating the focus or electroencephalographic change, but the behavior. Indeed, after surgery the patient will have—if we are speaking anatomically rather than functionally—a more damaged brain. Suppose we had an electroencephalographic change which correlated with increased intelligence, creativity, or sensitivity. No one would encourage operation on that "abnormality."

The "organic" model seems irrelevant and could lead to abuse in either direction. By implying the medical model it invites the kind of coercion and manipulation that the cure of organic illness invites. The organic label may be merely an amulet to comfort the surgeon by invoking the epileptic analogy. It is a false comfort, particularly when the only signs of equating the violent social behavior with epilepsy are the electroencephalographic changes (notoriously crude measuring instruments). Then again, in the opposite direction, psychiatrists are more than prepared to use organic therapies, e.g., drugs, to cure conditions such as depression or anxiety for which there is no well-defined, clearly demonstrable organic base. It would seem monstrous to restrict the use of those drugs to proven "organic" conditions. Organic versus functional is not the issue. The basic consideration should be the relative harmfulness of the procedure weighed against the impairments of the disease.

The Distinction Between Therapy and Social Control

There is every good reason why there has been a public outcry against surgery for the violence of temporal lobe epilepsy and not a similar one, for example, for the use of lithium in manic-depressive psychosis (an organic treatment for a disease with no demonstrable organic pathology). Beyond the distinction between surgery and drugs, which may well be exaggerated anyway, there is the distinction between an *intra*personal disease and an *inter*personal disease. With depression, the primary victim of the disease is the patient himself, and the primary beneficiary of the cure is the patient. He suffers both sets of consequences—from the illness and from the cure. With violent behavior, it is often the patient who pays the price of the procedure for benefits that are most directly felt by others.

That raises the frightening specter that under the guise of the beneficence of medicine, we are instituting another means of social control. This is not to rule out psychosurgery as a means of controlling violence. It is conceivable that *some* people in *some* societies might make a defensible case for this, but there can be no defense for confusing therapy and control, and disastrous consequences could issue by masking one under the other. It is understandable that some critics have raised serious questions as to the ultimate purpose of most psychosurgical research. The incidence of violent behavior directly linked to brain changes seems so low as to raise the question whether the ultimate uses of the extensive research being suggested are to cure illness or to seek controls of violence for social purposes. These speculations are given particular credence when as distinguished an authority as Dr. William H. Sweet will say in the introduction to *Violence and the Brain*: "While the ability to treat this special group of potentially violent persons represents only a small contribution to the solution of the total problem, it holds out the hope that knowledge gained about emotional brain function in violent persons with brain disease can be applied to combat the violence-triggering mechanisms in the brains of the nondiseased."[4]

Some of the extreme political rhetoric directed at psychosurgery suggests its potential utilization by a malevolent government. But electrode implantation or surgical ablation of brain sections as a direct means of political control seem unlikely—much less a threat, for example, than drugs. Such an individualized and dramatic procedure hardly seems suited to the enslavement of populations or the robotization of opposing political leaders. Drugs, brainwashing by control of the media, exploitation of fears through forms of propaganda, and indoctrination through the sources of education, particularly if preschool education or neonatal conditioning as suggested by Skinner becomes an approved practice, all seem more likely methods of totalitarian control.

This does not mean that we must not still be careful to draw a distinction between therapy and social control. All social control is not engineered through the political process or for national political purposes. There is no question that in mental institutions many devices that were proposed as therapeutic were utilized for purposes which were primarily custodial. They were intended not to benefit the patient but the staff, not to make the patient well but to make him manageable. This, too, must be recognized for what it is—a form of social control rather than therapy.

The Distinction Between Therapy and Social Engineering

When medicine moved into psychological and emotional aspects of behavior, a whole range of problems which were formerly not thought of as medical were introduced into the professional medical therapeutic way of thinking and assigned to certain rules of behavior which most of us accept as part of the medical contract. Without our realizing it, this medical contract sets conditions for behavior which are tacitly agreed upon by both the doers and those done to, often without either recognizing all that is happening. Much of what has been discussed in the preceding sections forms a part of the problems of this medical model. One particularly crucial aspect is the meaning of the concept of normalcy as used in medicine, and the confusion this creates when it is extended to neomedical or nonmedical conditions. In physiological functions normalcy is fairly easy to define and usually equatable with normative, i.e., good or, indeed, optimal. A temperature of 98.6°F. is normal in that it is the norm (average) for most of us, and in addition an ideal and optimal temperature. One could say the same thing for ten fingers or ten toes. Even with the physical there can be serious problems, however, although they do not warrant elaborate discussion here. "Low blood pressure," which had been considered a "disease" some years ago, represents one such confusion, and there are many more complex and subtle ones.

In mental health, however, the problems can be devastating. What is a "normal" attitude toward one's mother? What is a "normal" attitude toward work? Toward pleasure? Toward drugs? Toward pain? Not only confusion, but serious dangers to individual liberty are apparent when we start defining optimal behavior as a medically demandable norm. Certainly this can become a political device as expressed in its crudest form in the Medhvedev case in Russia.[5] Here the Soviets have demonstrated how mental institutions can be directly exploited to by-pass due process and judicial procedure. The stigmatization of insanity further discredits the dissenter.

But the coercive aspects of this concept of normalcy are more subtle and complex. It has been discussed elsewhere[3] and can only be summarized here. What is crucial is to realize that by changing the frame of reference under which we categorize a piece of behavior we create a potentially explosive and sociologically significant modification. We live in a culture that has always, at least theoretically, respected diversity in moral and religious areas, but which has granted to medicine certain rights to coercion. By redefining morality and values in medical terms, we are expanding the mechanism for controlling human behavior. By redefining a piece of behavior as abnormal rather than wrong, we are subjecting it to certain coercive aspects of law reserved for health issues.

Even without that we will have introduced certain covert coercive aspects. If a piece of behavior is defined as immoral by a religious authority, most individuals feel free to accept or reject that definition because our society endows religious moral leaders with little authority or punitive power. For the typical individual it is easier to change one's religion than to change a condemned but desired activity. If, however, a doctor defines the very same piece of behavior as "abnormal" or "sick," and if the individual is convinced of the doctor's expertise in matters of health—which is likely in our society—his own fear will force him to try to abandon that activity. More important, he will not feel forced; he will wish to do what the doctor wishes. The universal terror of illness, operating under the imprimatur of the medical establishment, will then make coercion in the traditional sense unnecessary. This is a potent force in behavior control which has not been nearly sufficiently analyzed, evaluated, or supervised.

Again, I suspect that in the areas of concern for manipulating man, social engineering will find direct intervention in the brain the least attractive of the mechanisms available. Certainly, conditioning at an early age is better suited for creating the "ideal" person. We all have a healthy revulsion against penetration of our innards, and surgically messing around with the brain has its own built-in controls in the aversive effect the very images present. In addition, it seems so final and irreversible a procedure that it will be shunned except as a procedure of last resort. To a psychiatrist, however, there is the certain knowledge that sensory inputs, particularly if initiated early in life, carry the fixity of organic change. If there is a difference between implanting an electrode and implanting an idea, it will require more elegant attention than it has as yet received.

Questions of Human Autonomy

In a recent behavior control meeting a distinguished brain researcher was describing the possibility of the humane use of implantation of electronic circuitry into the brain which could be controlled by an external box and would help manage impulsive behavior of an antisocial sort. After describing the miracle of the little box, he was asked if, once the effectiveness of the procedure had been secured, he would be willing to turn the box over to the patient. His answer was an immediate "Of course not." When asked "Why not?," he said, with the eloquence of simplicity, "It's my box."

Throughout the discussion in this chapter, human dignity and autonomy have been central, if not explicit, concerns. Perhaps the only essential wisdom in Dr. B. F. Skinner's book, *Beyond Freedom and Dignity*,[6] was the recognition that before massive extensive social engineering could be initiated, the concepts of both freedom and dignity must be attacked as not only dangerous, but false. Those of us who do not believe that they are false must be prepared to accept the dangers inherent in their reality— one of them being the real potential of the implementation, incrementally at least, of a controlling mankind in a controlled society.

Yet part of the uniqueness of man is the freedom to be that which we choose to be, even if "unfree." It is this peculiarity that accounts for the fact that in behavior control research, almost alone among all biological experimentation, success is more likely to breed dejection than joy. Devices that save or extend life aggrandize both the discoverer and man in general with the suggestion that such control of death, while still not the immortality of God, is a cut above the helplessness of the general animal host. Behavior manipulation, on the other hand, reasserts our kinship with the pigeon and the rat. The more technological the control devices, the more mechanical the method, the scarier it all seems. But to abandon our technology because of our fears would be an equal mistake. Technology can reduce man, but it has also enhanced him. To be afraid of our technology is to be afraid of ourselves. It is only essential that we protect ourselves here, as everywhere, from arrogance and insensitivity. The answer is not to prohibit technology but to insist that it always be subservient to the transcending values of human worth and human dignity.

REFERENCES

1. Breggin, Peter. "The Return of Lobotomy and Psychosurgery." *Congressional Record,* February 24, 1972, pp. E1602-E1612.

2. Freeman, Walter, and Watts, James. *Psychosurgery.* Springfield: Charles C. Thomas, 1942.

3. Gaylin, Willard. "On the Borders of Persuasion." *Psychiatry* 37(February 1974):1-9.

4. Mark, Vernon, and Ervin, Frank. *Violence and the Brain.* New York: Harper & Row, 1970, chap. 6.

5. Medhvedev, Zhores, and Medhvedev, Roy. *A Question of Madness.* New York: Knopf, 1971.

6. Skinner, B. F. *Beyond Freedom and Dignity.* New York: Knopf, 1971.

7. Snodgrass, Virginia. "Debate Over Benefits and Ethics of Psychosurgery Involves the Public." *Journal of American Medical Association* 225(August 20, 1973):913-920.

8. Veatch, Robert M. "Generalization of Expertise." *Hastings Center Studies* (1973):29-40.

HERBERT G. VAUGHAN, JR., M.D.

2 / Psychosurgery and Brain Stimulation in Historical Perspective

ALL CHANGES in experience or behavior are mediated through physiologic changes in the brain, whether induced by drugs, by conditioning, or by the more prosaic modes of education, persuasion, or physical coercion. Direct physical manipulation of the brain (PMB)—including removal or destruction of brain tissue or electrical or chemical stimulation—can be accorded a special status by virtue of its uniquely restricted use by a small professional elite, as well as the peculiar directness of effect which removes it from the subject's monitoring or control. Even drugs, which exert their psychological effects through their physiologic actions upon the brain, are less covert in their influence, since they are ordinarily openly administered and their effects are usually reversible. Thus to some degree the changes they produce in experience and behavior can be monitored and evaluated by the subject.

Destruction of brain tissue, when performed with the primary intent of modifying experience or behavior, can properly be called "psychosurgery," regardless of whether the procedure is carried out on a damaged or grossly normal brain.

Historically, psychosurgery was developed and applied in a strictly therapeutic context. It was viewed as a direct method for interrupting brain circuits which were thought to produce the

Library
I.U.P.
Indiana, Pa.
174.2 Op2e
c.1

severe emotional and behavioral disturbances associated with major psychosis. Psychosurgery has been performed on persons suffering from severe mental illnesses, the physiologic origins of which are little understood. Psychosurgical procedures have also been used to alter behavioral disturbances associated with overt brain damage, mainly, in retardates and epileptics. Since surgical brain destruction must have some cost in terms of reduced capacities, it is essential to define the nature and magnitude of the benefits to be gained from such procedures as well as the costs to be paid by the patient. These questions have existed since the earliest days of psychosurgery and, by and large, remain to be satisfactorily answered.

A fundamental concern regarding psychosurgery derives from its impact upon the personality—the idea that physical damage to the brain may be equated with destruction of the self. Questions of deep philosophic significance are raised by our growing understanding of the physiologic mechanisms that underlie human experience and behavior, and our increasing power to influence or control them. These must ultimately be dealt with in defining the acceptable place of psychosurgery and other potentially more selective techniques of physical brain manipulation in the armamentarium of psychiatric treatment.

To the extent that biological factors cause or contribute to psychic disturbances, efforts directed at modifying or eliminating pathological brain processes would appear to be valid modes of medical treatment. However, behavioral and emotional disorders always constitute an inextricable mixture of biological and psychosocial factors so that the notion of a purely biological approach to the treatment of mental illness is illusory. Although the search for biological causes of mental illness is essential for accomplishing the goal of preventing psychopathology associated with specific biologic abnormalities of brain function, the universality of biological etiologies cannot be assumed. The chain of evidence linking specific aspects of brain biology to mental illness is incomplete, and biological therapies are largely evaluated on a trial and error basis.

From the viewpoint of "biological psychiatry," which emphasizes the causal role of biologic brain dysfunction in mental illness,

25

the empirical search for effective biological therapies is a valid, indeed essential, component of the fight against mental illness. In contrast, those who emphasize the psychosocial aspects of psychopathology often tend to distrust, and may oppose on principle, therapeutic approaches which focus upon modifying the biological substrate of experience and behavior. This disparate explanatory base has rendered a dialogue on the pros and cons of psychosurgery virtually impossible.

The biological position is mainly a pragmatic one. Does it work? This viewpoint emphasizes the difficulties of environmental manipulation and the "failures" of primarily psychological methods of therapy. Such attitudes are favored in our highly competitive technological society and lead to pressures for simple biological "fixes" which are sought in all areas of medicine today.

Certainly, one could hardly find a broad consensus on what environmental modifications are needed, and in this setting the idea of dealing with behavioral deviance in the medical context, i.e., as conditions requiring treatment, is almost irresistible, as is evidenced by the redefinition of drug addiction and alcoholism as "diseases." We are now told that violent behavior can be due to brain pathology and may thus be amenable to surgical "treatment."

While it has been easy to sensationalize the grave deficiencies of psychosurgery as a therapeutic modality by emphasizing its drastic, irreversible, and unpredictable features, and capitalizing upon our seemingly inherent distaste for physical intrusion upon the brain, the problems posed by psychosurgery and other methods of PMB are far more subtle and complex than one might gather from recent discussions. To consider but one counterbalancing problem, what are the available or potential alternatives to psychosurgery in dealing with some of the more intractable forms of mental illness? It is becoming increasingly evident that drugs at present do not provide the hoped-for dramatic improvement in social recovery of psychotic patients, and are now seen to carry their own irreversible effects upon the brain. Many patients, both young and old, suffer from significant damage to brain structure which predisposes them to behavioral disorders. Institutionalization, combined with physical and pharmacological restraint, is often the dehumanizing fate of these unfortunate persons.

There are major unresolved therapeutic problems in psychiatry which are unlikely to be resolved without the most careful and intensive consideration of biological as well as psychosocial approaches. In the absence of suitable animal models of psychiatric illness, clinical investigation, both of mechanism and of therapeutic effectiveness and safety, will be required. Psychosurgery presents a particularly difficult problem of clinical evaluation, due to its irreversibility and the complexity of the psychobiological mechanisms it is intended to alter. The history of psychosurgery provides a prototype for considering the difficult issues posed by all unproven therapies which possess significant and often unknown risks.

Issues of a somewhat different nature are raised by the second major form of PMB: electrical stimulation of the brain (ESB), which has been employed as an important tool for the investigation of brain function for over a century, but the therapeutic potential of which has been recognized for less than a decade. There are several possible clinical applications of ESB, but attention has been most sharply focused on its potential for "shaping" behavior under the control of the operator by using intracranial stimulation as a reward or "positive reinforcer." ESB has barely moved beyond the realm of science fiction, but already serious concerns have been expressed regarding the possibility of legally or morally questionable application.

Although psychosurgery and ESB are both classified as techniques for physical brain manipulation, their mode of action, their therapeutic potential, and their dangers differ strikingly. Psychosurgery destroys brain tissue, and thus in the physical sense is an irreversible procedure, whereas ESB (and the intracranial application of neuroactive chemicals) is nondestructive and usually reversible in its immediate effects. The effects of psychosurgery are subtractive and largely impossible to predict in terms of specific behavioral changes. Its therapeutic potential derives from a reduction of unpleasant or maladaptive affect, permitting the patient to redirect his activities. Thus psychosurgery does not "control" behavior, but produces behavioral changes which are secondary to modification of emotional mechanisms.

27

The untoward effects of psychosurgery seem to derive mainly from undesirable changes in motivation and reduced self-consciousness concerning the social significance of the patient's own behavior. In contrast, ESB and chemostimulation operate through neural mechanisms by temporarily activating or inhibiting their action. These techniques can alter feelings in a definable way. If fear or pleasure are systematically elicited by ESB in association with specific situations or behaviors, permanent alterations in emotional and behavioral responses can be achieved, in accordance with well-established principles of learning. These changes could be under the control of a therapist, the person himself, or any operator who controls the stimulating apparatus. The obvious possibilities for misuse of these potent techniques have led some to question the desirability of further experimentation in this area and to doubt the wisdom of any therapeutic application of ESB or chemostimulation. Yet a great therapeutic advantage could be gained from such nondestructive and highly specific methods over inherently destructive and less predictable methods of psychosurgery, and even over presently available psychoactive drugs. Furthermore, there is an important potential for the treatment of epilepsy and in prosthetic applications, which employ a common technology with the psychological application of ESB but do not pose the hazard of behavior control.

All of the present techniques for PMB derive ultimately from experimental studies of the brain mechanisms which underlie experience and behavior. Much of this work has been done in animals, but a good many critical observations, especially regarding the role of the brain in conscious experience, have of necessity been made in man. The history of neurosurgery presents an admixture of bold therapeutic innovation combined with observations essentially motivated by scientific curiosity. Information derived from the latter has often provided a critical ingredient of the former. Those who have devoted themselves to the search for means to ameliorate neurologic and psychiatric disorders through a direct attack upon their underlying mechanisms have recognized and emphasized, often to the exclusion of other considerations, the need to understand brain mechanisms more fully in order to achieve safe and effective therapeutic measures. There is, however, a critical need to consider all of the relevant scientific, clinical, social, and ethical factors in depth as a prerequisite for defining a humane course of basic investigation and therapeutic experimentation in the area of PMB.

The Experimental Background of Psychosurgery— The Effects of Brain Lesions on Behavior

The brain was first identified as the seat of human experience and behavior over 25 centuries ago, when inferences on relationships between brain function and psychological processes were derived from the natural experiments of disease and trauma. It was the behavioral effects of brain wounds inflicted in battle and the manifestations of epileptic brain discharges which pointed to the brain as the physical substrate of sensation, thought, volition, and emotion. Little direct evidence on the anatomic representation of these various psychic functions within the brain was then available.

Despite the paucity of specific information on brain-behavior correlations, surgical intrusion into the brain was well known by the time of the Hippocratic writings in the fourth century B.C. Indeed, prehistoric evidence of trephination has been found in both old and new world skulls, indicating the early and widespread practice of cranial surgery for purposes which remain entirely unknown. These findings suggest that even prehistoric man may have possessed some appreciation of the role of the brain in mental functions. During the centuries which followed the decay of Greco-Roman civilization, much biological knowledge was lost or perverted with the general decline in intellectual life which characterized the Middle Ages. Hippocratic notions concerning the physiologic basis of mental activity were supplanted by mystical conceptions of the human mind which were ultimately embodied in Descartes's distinction between mental and biological processes. The Cartesian doctrine formalized the dichotomy of mind and brain which still influences much contemporary thinking, even among biologists.

Interest in the nervous system was rekindled with the resurgence in active investigations of natural phenomena which

29

accompanied the Renaissance. A series of experimental studies demonstrated the fundamental properties of irritability and conductivity which characterize nervous tissue, and established the electrical nature of nerve action. The anatomy of the brain was studied and the basic structural similarities among mammalian brains noted. During the eighteenth and nineteenth centuries neurobiological studies proceeded in many areas and, as in the age of Greek medicine, observations on the effects of brain diseases provided important information on the physiologic basis of psychologic processes. By the late 1800s postmortem observations on the location of brain damage had been compared with symptoms occurring during life, and the broad outlines of specific representation of sensory, motor, and language processes within the human brain had emerged.

These nineteenth-century students of brain function did not limit their observations to behavioral disorders due to cerebral disease. Experimental approaches employing selective surgical excisions were employed to define more precisely the functional role of specific cerebral regions. These studies were carried out in a wide variety of animals, including birds, dogs, and, ultimately, several primate species. The investigation of human patients with cerebral disease and of experimental lesions in animals complemented one another; the human studies were often deficient in knowledge of the anatomical extent of the brain lesions, which were determined by the vagaries of disease rather than the requirements for precise anatomical analysis. Even when the pathology could be defined postmortem, the disease process had often changed the condition of the brain between the clinical observations and final anatomical examination. The opportunity to perform well-defined surgical excisions of brain tissue provided a necessary complement to the human studies, but the difficulty of analyzing behavioral changes in experimental animals, together with the differences in brain structure and behavior between man and even his closer primate relations, limited the application to man of experimental animal neuropsychology.

It is important to understand the problems and limitations of animal investigations, since these comprise the approach, short of experimentation on human patients, through which knowledge of the behavioral effects of brain manipulation can be obtained. A critical view of such animal studies is required, since these have often been cited to justify the clinical application of a particular surgical procedure, sometimes without a full appreciation of their inadequacies.

An important limitation of animal studies derives from the inability of the subjects to communicate their experiences verbally. Although behaviorists discount the value of "subjective" report, lack of evidence on how the subject "feels" and how he regards a particular situation or task often poses difficult and sometimes insuperable obstacles to the interpretation of complex behavior, and obviously precludes an insight into the animal's actual experiences. Behavioral psychologists have dealt with these issues either by ignoring them or by redefining experiential variables in terms of behavior. This has led to ambiguities and unwarranted assumptions concerning the processes within the animal brain which actually lead to a given behavior. Especially in the crucial area of affect and motivation, serious difficulties are encountered in interpretation of experimental effects.

For example, a rat's ability to avoid a foot shock can be altered by placing lesions in certain brain areas,[21] but it has required the most elaborate experiments to define the mechanisms by which the animal becomes more or less responsive to a "painful" shock. Is pain perception altered? Is the resultant emotional response modified? Or is the change in avoidance behavior related to motor effects? Surprisingly, differences in appreciation of pain or an emotional response may not account for the changes in avoidance behavior, since by using different tests—one requiring an "escape" to avoid shock (active avoidance) and the other the *inhibition* of a motor activity (passive avoidance)—opposite effects on "avoidance behavior" can be produced by the same brain lesion. In this instance the initiation of motor activity is affected by the lesion—perhaps the least obvious interpretation of the original observations. Thus one lesson to be derived from animal neuropsychology is that great caution must be exercised in making inferences about animal experience from behavioral observations.

There are additional complexities in the effects of brain lesions upon human as well as animal behavior. First, a circumscribed brain lesion does not often produce simple effects on behavior. Early observations on behavioral changes following brain damage focused upon those which were most prominent and easiest to define. Attention was first paid to motor and sensory effects. Once the rather gross impairments of movement and sensory capacity were defined, it was necessary to develop more refined techniques of behavioral analysis. These tests, while more precise, focus upon more limited areas of behavior. Experimental neuropsychology has developed these techniques to a high degree during recent decades, so that precise methods for evaluating deficiencies in perceptual organization and in some cognitive functions are now available. Studies using these methods in experimental animals subjected to local brain lesions have partially defined the role of specific brain areas in a number of rather complex psychological processes, such as visual perception. Although roughly parallel neuropsychological studies have been carried out in human patients with various kinds of brain damage, the nature and results of the animal and human studies have often not been comparable. Consequently, there is presently some lack of congruence between the experimental and clinical investigations, even in the best-studied areas of sensory and perceptual functioning. When one turns to the more complex areas of cognitive function and emotional behavior, the situation is even more difficult. Even though most of our knowledge in this area is confounded by the prominent species differences among the major experimental subjects—rats, cats, and primates—certain general themes can be extracted from the body of experimental results.

In contrast to the effects of small removals of cortical tissue which may produce distinct sensory or motor deficits, the appearance of gross disorders of complex behavior requires either very large cortical lesions or smaller lesions which involve deep brain areas. The classical experimental demonstrations of the effects of large cerebral lesions were made on frontal lobe damage in monkeys by Bianchi[2] and on bilateral temporal lobectomy by Klüver and Bucy.[19] Removals of either the frontal or the temporal lobes produced major changes in the behavior of monkeys, but

without the severe motor and/or sensory deficits which characterized lesions of the central and posterior parts of the cerebral
hemispheres. Although differing substantially in their overall
behavioral effects, both the frontal and temporal lobe removals
produced a major impairment in adaptive capacities, with disruption of the monkey's usual behavior and inappropriate responses
to the environment. The frontal lobe lesions were characterized by
indifference to objects of previous interest. Social behavior was
disrupted, and normal expressions of affection or aversion
blunted. Yet the monkeys remained capable of emotional responses when directly confronted with appropriate stimuli. These
responses might even be exaggerated, but they possessed a passive
character and were terminated when attention was shifted to a
new stimulus. The emotional changes described by Bianchi were
not stereotyped, but appeared characteristic of each animal. Such
changes have been interpreted by later workers as exaggerations of
the monkeys' preoperative personality. This work showed that
observations of the monkey's general behavior before and after
surgery made it possible to detect changes in personality and
general adaptive abilities which are not disclosed by the more
precise and focused behavioral tests employed in more recent
studies.

The observations of Klüver and Bucy on monkeys after bilateral
temporal lobectomy revealed extraordinary behavioral changes
which included a striking loss of fear responses, hypersexuality,
and a peculiar inability to recognize familiar objects visually,
although basic visual functions appeared to be intact. The
behavioral effects of these extensive lesions are very complicated,
and scientists have dissected these disturbances into components
associated with the functions of smaller regions within the frontal
and temporal lobes. These efforts were consonant with the
concept of functional localization within the brain which had,
with some exceptions, been dominant in neuropsychology since
the mid-nineteenth century.

However, studies of experimental ablations led to opposing
concepts of brain organization. In the eighteenth century Pierre
Flourens, working with birds, and in the twentieth century Karl
Lashley,[20] working largely with rats, espoused the notion that

behavior derives from the integrated activity of the entire brain, and that local lesions exert their effects mainly by reducing the overall effectiveness of brain functioning. These ideas, known as the theory of "equipotentiality," were strongly championed by Lashley on the basis of observations on complex maze-learning behavior. In contrast, those who studied the effects of brain lesions in man tended to favor the alternative notion which emphasized regional differences in functional organization of the brain. In their extreme form, these "localizationist" views deteriorated into the absurd mosaic ideas of brain organization propounded by phrenologists. The truth, as is so often the case, falls somewhere between the extreme localizationalist and equipotentialist views. Modern neuropsychology acknowledges the fact that behavior is dependent upon the integrated functioning of extensive brain areas, but recognizes the specialization of brain regions or systems for particular aspects of behavior.

These functional systems seem to be quite circumscribed in some instances when defined by the behavioral effects of a localized lesion. But often what is being demonstrated is the destruction of a *necessary* component of a more extensive system. For example, loss of consciousness can be produced by a very small lesion in a critical site within the upper portion of the brain stem which connects the cerebral hemispheres to the spinal cord. But it is meaningless to impute the function of "consciousness" to this region, since the cerebral hemispheres are also involved in the processes underlying conscious experience. Similarly, paralysis of the hand may be produced by removing a circumscribed area of the cerebral cortex. This effectively interrupts the brain mechanisms underlying normal movement control, which, however, also involve other brain regions.

Conversely, a brain lesion may appear to produce little or no behavioral deficit, but may nevertheless affect the functional capacity of the individual when placed under stress. It seems that the human brain possesses a great deal more potential, especially in the more complex areas of cognitive function, than is employed in most activities of life. This situation apparently accounts for the relatively slight impact of large frontal lobe lesions on formally tested intelligence. Only when the person is challenged to make new adaptations or to develop new ways of thinking does the intellectual deficiency produced by frontal lobe lesions become manifest. Because of these and other complexities yet to be discussed, the analysis of functions of regions within the frontal and temporal cortex has proceeded slowly and laboriously and rests to a large extent on the results of experimental studies in monkeys.

Since Jacobsen's[18] early observations on specific behavioral disturbance following selective frontal cortex lesions, many studies have attempted to identify the nature of psychological processes represented in various parts of the frontal cortex. Such studies have even been carried out in man. One of the studies of psychosurgery by the Columbia-Greystone Associates in the late 1940s[3] assessed the effects of localized cortical removals (topectomy) on the symptoms and psychological functioning of a series of psychiatric patients. By and large, however, these studies have led to few generalizations applicable to the understanding of human frontal lobe function. Indeed, in the recent words of an eminent neuropsychologist, the frontal lobes remain a riddle after almost a century of study.[42]

It is an extraordinary fact that an almost casual observation by Jacobsen and Fulton,[11] on a single monkey's emotional behavior following frontal lobe lesioning, formed the entire empirical basis for the proposal of the frontal lobotomy as a psychiatric treatment—a procedure which has been carried out on perhaps 50,000 persons since 1935. It is hardly surprising that the early psychosurgery, carried out in such ignorance of the great complexity and subtlety of frontal lobe mechanisms, should have led to serious and sometimes disabling psychological side effects which ultimately brought all surgical approaches to psychiatric treatment into widespread disrepute.

At present, it is possible to separate frontal lobe functions into two broad categories having distinct anatomical substrates—those processes which are related to attention and to the initiation and inhibition of motor activity, including speech, which are mainly affected by lesions involving the superior and lateral cortical areas; and those related to drives and autonomic nervous system functions which are intimately concerned with emotion and

35

motivation. These latter functions are primarily represented in the cortex on the under surface of the frontal lobes. This region is in close anatomical relation to the hypothalamus and other portions of the limbic system which are discussed below. Current psychosurgical approaches to the frontal lobes emphasize the therapeutic effects of lesions which interrupt the connections of orbital and medial cortex, thus reducing unpleasant and disabling emotional responses while sparing the dorsolateral connections which mediate processes important for sustained attention and cognitive function.

The temporal lobes present functional aspects as complicated as those of the frontal areas. It has again been possible to distinguish between functions of the lateral temporal cortex, which are mainly concerned with auditory, sensory and perceptual analysis, and processes mediated by the medial and deep structures, which are related to emotion—and surprisingly to learning and memory. Many experimental studies of localized lesions within the temporal lobe followed the description of the Klüver-Bucy syndrome.[19] Although most of these have been done in monkeys, one exceedingly important observation was made in man—in this case, an unexpected and serious complication of a psychosurgical experiment. Scoville,[38] seeking an alternative to frontal lobe surgery, reasoned that removal of areas within the temporal lobe which received anatomic projections from the orbital frontal region might prove effective. Accordingly, he performed bilateral excisions of the medial portion of the temporal lobes in 30 "severely deteriorated" schizophrenic patients and one patient with intractable epileptic seizures. Although the patients showed no improvement in the condition for which they were operated, and no apparent deterioration of general intellectual functioning, it was found that eight patients, in whom the excisions included the hippocampus on both sides showed a moderate to severe impairment of recent memory. This deficit has been intensively studied in the nonpsychotic epileptic patient by psychologist Brenda Milner.[27] It apparently reflects a critical role of the hippocampal region of the temporal lobes in the process of learning. Curiously, it has not been possible to demonstrate a comparable memory defect in subsequent efforts to duplicate this effect by experimental hippocampal lesions in monkeys. This circumstance serves as a further warning concerning the application to man of neuropsychological studies in animals.

It may be representative of widespread attitudes within the medical profession that despite the extraordinary interest generated by the report of these findings[38] virtually no comment was made upon the circumstance that 30 patients had been subjected to a previously untried and potentially hazardous psychosurgical procedure before the existence of a severe psychological deficit was discovered. This incident would seem, at the very least, to have dictated the most stringent care in psychological evaluation of patients subjected to any removal or destruction of brain tissue. Yet the clinical literature since that time contains little evidence that such precautions are routinely taken by practitioners of psychosurgery.

The most important insights into the neurological substrate of emotional behavior derive from studies of the effects of lesions deep within the brain substance. Bard[1] showed in 1928 that tame cats manifested vicious behavior at the slightest provocation when all of the brain, except a tiny region at its base, called the hypothalamus, was disconnected from the lower parts of the nervous system. Extensive investigations have since been made of the neural basis of aggressive and other forms of emotional behavior in experimental animals. In no other area of neuropsychology have all of the experimental techniques available to the neuroscientist been more effectively coordinated, with the study of lesions, electrical stimulation, neuroanatomy, and neuropharmacology all contributing to an increasingly complete but extraordinarily complicated picture of the neural control of emotional behavior and related psychobiological processes.

These studies have emphasized the role of a group of interconnected structures, lying deep within the cerebral hemispheres and at the base of the brain, which are often designated the "limbic system." Among the main groups of nerve cells comprising this system are the hippocampus and amygdala, both located within the temporal lobe; the septal region and hypothalamus, at the base of the brain; and the anterior thalamic nuclei and cingulate gyri in the central portions of the cerebral hemispheres. These structures are interconnected with each other as well as with other cortical and subcortical regions. Within the limbic system there are important regional specializations, with different and often opposing forms of emotional behavior being represented within adjacent or even overlapping areas. It is now well established that the emotional aspects of limbic system function are closely integrated with the endocrine and autonomic nervous system activities associated with specific forms of emotional behavior. Thus areas which are concerned with the control of sexual behavior are not only sensitive to the sex hormones but are themselves involved in regulating the secretion of these hormones.[23]

The functional manifestations of the systems which control emotional behavior are subject to important environmental influences which include direct sensory experiences as well as indirect effects mediated by the actions of hormones upon the brain. Effects of limbic system lesions, and of other damaged brain structures as well, are often dependent upon the particular environmental circumstances in which the animal is tested. These effects are especially prominent in relation to drive-related behaviors—such as aggression and sexual activity—a circumstance which may have critical significance for the use of psychosurgery to modify violent behavior or sexual deviance.

In addition to the modifying effects of the environment on the psychological changes associated with brain lesions, attention must be paid to the occurrence of substantial anatomical overlap of systems subserving different psychological mechanisms, and also to the striking capacities often shown for recovery of function following brain lesions, in considering the use of brain lesions for therapeutic purposes. From a strictly anatomical standpoint, brain systems are rarely segregated from one another, even in regions such as the hypothalamus, wherein tiny lesions of adjacent areas may produce widely diverse effects. If the cellular architecture of the brain is examined by methods which show the full ramification of nerve cell processes rather than just their bodies, one can readily appreciate that a given focal lesion, if it involves cellular collections such as the cortex or the deep brain nuclei must damage the neural connections of regions surrounding the actual lesion for some distance. This may be one reason why several behavioral mechanisms are often affected by a local brain lesion. For example, experimental lesions of the amygdala, which is the target of one psychosurgical procedure, may not only produce a taming or "anti-aggressive" effect but hypersexuality and changes in hormonal secretions of the pituitary gland as well. The full behavioral ramifications of a specific brain lesion often become clear only after long and arduous experimental analysis, especially when the effects are not manifested by gross behavioral changes.

It has long been recognized that some forms of behavior can show marked recovery following their loss due to a brain lesion. This capacity often permits the rehabilitation of patients who have suffered from a stroke or other brain insult. Experimental studies have shown that such recovery may be mediated in part by the expression of functional capacities in brain areas which had not previously been actively involved in these processes. For example, lesioning of a particular hypothalamic site in the rat will cause the animal to refuse food and water, although his behavior seems to be normal in other respects.[41] If not tube-fed, he will soon die. However, if his life is sustained by forced feeding he will eventually begin to eat and drink, finally showing full recovery. Should an additional hypothalamic lesion then be inflicted in an adjacent site which would not affect feeding behavior in a normal rat, the aphagia will recur. It appears that the newly lesioned hypothalamic area had taken over the functions of the previously destroyed feeding center. Just as normal mechanisms may recover following brain lesions, the pathologic systems suppressed by psychosurgery may recur following an initial period of remission. The plasticity of brain mechanisms cannot be ignored in assessing the permanence of behavioral changes produced by brain lesions, a circumstance which precludes a simple conceptualization of either the favorable or the untoward effects of psychosurgery.

The Rise and Decline of Frontal Lobotomy

Frontal lobotomy, the first rational attempt to ameliorate symptoms of severe mental illness by surgical methods, was proposed by Portuguese neurologist Egas Moniz in 1935. In that year the experiments of Fulton and Jacobsen on the behavioral effects of frontal lobe lesions in monkeys were reported at the International Congress of Neurology in London. These workers commented on the resistance of one of their lesioned monkeys to the "experimental neurosis" ordinarily associated with failure in their testing situation. In the ensuing discussion, Moniz reasoned that a similar effect might be obtained upon the emotional distress and obsessive rumination of patients suffering from mental illness, and proposed the therapeutic sectioning of the subcortical connections of the frontal lobes. With the neurosurgeon Almeida Lima he devised methods for severing the connections between the cortex of the frontal lobe and the underlying thalamic nuclei, first using injections of alcohol and later a cutting device which removed a small sphere of subcortical tissue. Twenty patients in a mental hospital near Lisbon were operated on within a brief period, and the results of the procedure reported within the year.[28] The apparently favorable effects of the surgery on the majority of these severely disturbed patients led to its introduction in the U.S. by neurologist Walter Freeman and his surgical colleague James Watts. Until his recent death, Freeman remained the foremost American protagonist of frontal lobotomy, having over 3,500 cases in his personal experience.

From the outset, psychosurgical procedures aroused strong emotions among advocates and detractors. Before 1945, however, lobotomy seemed to make little impact upon psychiatric treatment. Fewer than 1,000 operations had been performed in the United States since its introduction ten years earlier. From 1945 to 1950, however, there was a veritable explosion in the use of frontal lobotomy, which reached a peak of 5,000 operations per year in 1949. According to assertions made at the time, the extraordinary postwar acceleration in the use of psychosurgery occurred in response to "public pressures" for more effective treatment of mentally ill war veterans. The popularity of lobotomy was further enhanced by Freeman's introduction of the transorbital technique. This method, which required no conventional surgical opening of the skull but only a quick thrust of a specially designed instrument through the thin bony roof of the orbit, opened the performance of lobotomy to the entire medical profession. Indeed, these "icepick" lobotomies were so simple to perform that Freeman advocated their use by general physicians. Although resisted by neurosurgeons, the technique rapidly achieved extensive use in sections of the country which possessed limited surgical resources. The transorbital procedure involved a less radical destruction of frontal lobe connections and, in Freeman's experience, actually possessed a lower rate of morbidity and mortality than the "standard" lobotomy procedures which required surgical opening of the skull. The extent to which the transorbital method took hold remains uncertain, although figures compiled by NIMH[34] indicate that fully one-third of all lobotomies employed the transorbital method in 1949, three years after its introduction. It is of interest that no transorbital lobotomies were done in New England, a region with substantial neurosurgical resources, whereas in the West South Central region (Texas, Oklahoma, Arkansas, and Louisiana) 90 percent of lobotomies used this technique. The striking regional variations in method and in the overall number of operations at that time suggest that factors other than therapeutic effectiveness influenced the selection of treatment for severe mental illness.

The major expansion in the use of lobotomy between 1945 and 1949 occurred before any organized effort was made to assess the therapeutic effects of the procedure beyond the experience of individual psychiatrists and psychosurgeons. By 1949, however, several intensive studies of psychosurgery had been mounted, with the Columbia-Greystone projects[3,4] and the studies carried out at the Boston Psychopathic Hospital[13] being among the best-known. Most of these studies supported the notion that lobotomy performed on patients who had failed to respond to other available treatments carried with it a more favorable outcome than the institutional management then current. Furthermore, despite the occurrence of major untoward effects on personality in some instances, these studies disclosed little or no evidence of intellectual deterioration following surgery. The rate of hospital discharge substantially exceeded that which might have been expected, especially since the patients selected for surgery in these studies were often chronic institutionalized schizophrenics. There were few claims of "cures," but reductions in anxiety, tension, and depression occurred in many patients. The delusions of schizophrenics seemed largely unaltered, but these were a matter of less concern to the patient.

The therapeutic effects of lobotomy were clearly linked to a reduction of unpleasant affect and did little to alter coexisting thought disorders. It became increasingly evident that the therapeutic results of lobotomy were closely related to the level of premorbid social adjustment, with a high level of performance permitting a quite favorable outcome. Freeman cited instances in which successful professional careers had been pursued postlobotomy.[9] However, these cases appear to number but a handful among his several thousand.

The extensive literature on psychosurgery which appeared during the late 1940s and 1950s documented in some detail both the favorable and untoward effects of frontal lobotomy. Wide variations in thoroughness and in methodology, together with the difficulties inherent in description and classification of psychiatric disorders, make it difficult to arrive at firm general conclusions concerning either the quality of therapeutic effects or the incidence and severity of unfavorable personality changes after surgery. The severity of the classical "frontal lobe syndrome" (loss of initiative, inappropriate joviality, and social insensitivity) which occurred in many patients following lobotomy was apparently directly related to the therapeutic reduction of anxiety, so that a truly satisfactory result represented a tenuous balance between failure to achieve any effect and unacceptable personality change. Considerable efforts were made both to refine the diagnostic criteria, which would improve the incidence of successful results, as well as to further surgical experimentation intended to limit the untoward personality deficits through less extensive sectioning of frontal lobe connections. Unfortunately, interest in the detailed follow-up and clinical study of patients who had received psychosurgical treatment waned sharply along with the use of lobotomy after the early 1950s, so that adequate long-term studies are virtually nonexistent, although a few inconclusive and somewhat conflicting reports have appeared.

Despite the relative simplicity of the frontal lobotomy, whether the transorbital variety or the standard surgical approach, and the apparently salutary effects of the procedure in a majority of patients, the use of lobotomy reached a high point in 1949 and showed slight decreases over the succeeding 18-month period (after which no published figures are available). Although there is a popular belief that the introduction of psychoactive drugs was the main factor in the decline of psychosurgery, the evidence suggests that use of the method may have declined even before the widespread use of antipsychotic drugs in the mid-1950s. It is important to know just what factors did operate during the period 1950-1955 to determine the selection of psychiatric treatment for severely disturbed patients. Although the series of conferences on psychosurgery sponsored by the NIMH between 1949 and 1951[34,35,36] clearly documented the general inadequacy of clinical evaluation and reporting on the treatment of psychiatric disorders, these critical issues were not intensively pursued in subsequent years and appeared largely forgotten by the time that large-scale use of antipsychotic drugs began to make possible extensive reductions in the population of public institutions for the mentally ill.

Contemporary Psychosurgery

While frontal lobotomy fell into disuse as a major treatment for mental illness during the 1950s, a number of neurosurgeons continued to perform these operations, trying to devise technical modifications which would increase the specificity of therapeutic results and diminish the untoward personality effects which so often accompanied the classical lobotomies. It is rather difficult to evaluate the psychosurgical activities of the past two decades, since the literature, while copious, continues to report inadequately the critical clinical details concerning the indication and outcome of the various procedures. An overview of the scope of this work up to 1970 is provided in *Psychosurgery: Proceedings of the Second International Conference.*[17] The conceptual basis provided by several of the more inventive practitioners for the continuing experimentation is not very edifying. Most of the efforts to modify the standard lobotomy have experimented with somewhat more limited sections of frontal lobe fibers in an attempt to define the "critical" sites for a therapeutic effect. The results have not been entirely consistent, but the relative efficacy of inferior and medial lesions for altering affective disturbances without serious personality deficits is emphasized.

In evaluating the literature, one must constantly try to read between the lines concerning the actual clinical experiences which have led psychosurgeons to be dissatisfied with one procedure and to try constantly to improve upon their operations. It is by no means clear that psychiatric, rather than technical, considerations have guided the pressures for innovation. The atmosphere in which psychosurgery has been carried out during the past two decades has made proper clinical evaluation extraordinarily difficult. Generally, the procedures are done either by individual practitioners or in the relatively few psychiatric institutions which remain committed to psychosurgical treatment. Often the clinical evaluations seem to have been made by the surgeons themselves, or by psychologists or social workers whose psychiatric training and competence is often unclear. The suspicion and hostility among the advocates and opponents of psychosurgery make unbiased comparative evaluations of treatment difficult, if not impossible.

The problem of therapeutic evaluation is not, however, limited to psychosurgery, but is a matter of general concern for psychiatry. Although the defensiveness and hostility which plagues the assessment of psychosurgery is not a major factor in the evaluation of psychoactive drugs, the serious difficulties in evaluating their therapeutic effectiveness are common to the evaluation of all of the somatic and psychotherapeutic approaches to the treatment of mental illness. It is unfortunate that an issue of such great importance has been so ineffectively dealt with, despite the enormous resources which have been expended on the delivery of care for the mentally ill. The fact that assessment of therapy in mental illness, especially in institutional settings, is generally deficient must be kept in mind when considering the special problems which face the evaluation of psychosurgery from the standpoint of safety and effectiveness.

Despite the unsatisfactory situation regarding therapeutic evaluation, substantial efforts have been made among a small group of neurosurgeons* to devise new techniques and to evaluate new lesion sites for the treatment of an increasingly broad array of psychiatric and behavioral disorders. The major technical innovation which has made much of this surgical experimentation possible is the stereotaxic method of producing brain lesions. This technique has made it possible to reach virtually any location within the brain with recording, stimulating, and lesioning probes. Methods have also been devised for cooling the brain to produce a reversible depression of function, and for introducing tiny amounts of neuroactive chemicals into specific brain sites. These techniques provide potent tools for the analysis and modification of brain function, and have been extensively employed in animal experimentation. During the past 25 years the development and application of these methods to clinical situations has brought about revolutionary new capabilities for what may be called "functional neurosurgery."

Neurosurgeons have been active in attempts to deal with a number of disorders which do not fall within the area of psychopathology and thus have been outside the scope of "psychosurgery." Other applications of functional neurosurgery include the treatment of intractable pain, epilepsy, and movement disorders, such as Parkinsonism and dystonia. These endeavors share with psychosurgery the rationale of attempting to ameliorate a particular abnormal symptom or behavior by lesioning a brain region considered necessary for the expression of the particular abnormality. In these instances the lesion is designed to interrupt the abnormal physiologic mechanisms which are responsible for the clinical abnormality. The tissue to be destroyed is not necessarily pathological. Selection of a specific lesion site is guided by knowledge of the anatomical pathways which constitute a

---

*It has been estimated that less than 5 percent of U.S. neurosurgeons perform psychosurgical procedures. Only a handful can be identified by published reports as active practitioners and innovators in the field.

45

particular functional brain system. Thus the surgical treatment for chronic pain involves either the sectioning of the nerve fibers carrying pain information to the brain, or of certain areas of the brain which experimental studies have implicated in the appreciation of pain.

Often several different lesions have been tried out on patients before a satisfactory result has been obtained. It is interesting that relatively little public complaint has been directed against therapeutic experiments directed to the surgical treatment of pain and movement disorders. It is possible that some of the differences in attitude concerning psychosurgery and other applications of functional neurosurgery can be related to distinctions, made by the public and the medical profession alike, concerning the nature of the disorders being treated. For example, chronic pain and motor disorders such as Parkinsonism are viewed as "organic" or "neurological" conditions for which selective interference with brain function seems appropriate, whereas psychopathology, being a derangement of the mind, poses difficulties for the acceptance of treatment directed against the underlying brain mechanisms. Although the force of the conceptual dichotomy between mind and brain has been substantially reduced by evidence demonstrating the dependence of mental processes upon brain mechanisms, willful alteration of the personality of a human being through the slash of a knife or a stereotaxic lesion represents to many a direct intrusion upon the most private aspects of the self—essentially, an assault upon the soul.

Surgical treatment of epilepsy presents a special case of particular importance for the present discussion, since both the classic surgical rationale of removing pathologic tissue and the approach of functional surgery, which attacks a pathophysiologic mechanism without regard to the presence of structural abnormality in the lesioned tissues, are employed. The surgical treatment of epilepsy developed by Penfield[31] was directed toward the identification and removal of a localized brain abnormality, usually a superficial scar of the cerebral cortex resulting from a penetrating head injury. It was also known from clinical observations supplemented by electroencephalography that the "psychomotor" form of epilepsy, often associated with seizures having complex behavioral and psychic manifestations, emanated from damaged tissue deep within the temporal lobes. Following the rationale employed in treating superficial cortical scars, the entire anterior part of the temporal lobe was resected; however, in this case it was necessary to remove normal brain along with the diseased tissue. At first it was thought that this could be done with impunity, as long as the visual pathways and language areas located in the more posterior part of the temporal lobe were spared. However, Brenda Milner[27] found that unilateral temporal lobectomy did produce subtle defects in perceptual and language functioning. Bilateral lobectomy produced the disastrous memory loss which had been inadvertently discovered in Scoville's efforts to improve upon the frontal lobotomy. Therefore, the fairly common problem of patients with bilateral temporal epileptic foci could not safely be treated by temporal lobectomy. In these instances, some surgeons thought that stereotaxic lesioning of the amygdala, often the site of epileptic discharge, might produce a therapeutic effect on the seizures while avoiding damage to the neighboring hippocampus, whose removal seemed to be responsible for the memory defect, and to the overlying cortex, implicated in perceptual and language mechanisms.

At this point a convergence between psychosurgery and the surgical treatment of epilepsy occurred. Japanese neurosurgeon Narabayashi, who was also a pioneer in the treatment of Parkinsonism by stereotaxic surgery, introduced the stereotaxic amygdalotomy as a means of managing hyperactive and violent children.[29] This procedure was based on the observed taming effect in naturally aggressive animals through bilateral lesioning of the amygdala. The children in whom this procedure was employed were severely brain-damaged and often epileptic as well, but the operation was specifically designed to curb their distressing behavior. Thus was born what is now the most controversial application of psychosurgery—the management of violent aggressive behavior.

The Surgery of Violence

Application of psychosurgical methods to the management of aggressive and violent behavior grew out of the vexing problem posed by the behavioral disturbances commonly encountered in children and adults suffering from severe brain damage. Erratic assaults upon others and self-mutilations are familiar incidents in institutions for the aged, the retarded, and the mentally ill. Indeed, the frontal lobotomy in its heyday had been advocated for the management of some of these problems. Amygdalotomy, however, appeared to provide a more specific antidote to aggressive outbursts. In the United States such patients are generally hidden from view in various institutions, so that pressures for medical management beyond the heavy use of tranquilizing drugs have not been great. In contrast, cultural circumstance in Japan has provided a strong motivation for more effective management of aggressive brain-damaged children, so as to permit them to be cared for in the home.[37] Institutionalization of a child there is associated with severe social stigma, so even severely retarded and brain-damaged children are maintained at home to the limits of the family's tolerance. It is alleged that family suicides have occurred under the stress of these circumstances. The introduction of amygdalotomy by Narabayashi and the posterior hypothalamotomy by Sano was supposedly intended to permit such hyperactive and destructive children to remain under the care of their families.

The exact indications and results of this "sedative surgery" are not readily apparent from the published reports of these several hundred operations on children, nor have the descriptions of the much smaller number of operations performed in the U.S. been enlightening. This work received virtually no public attention until the use of amygdalotomy for the management of violent behavior achieved notoriety through the publication of *Violence and the Brain* by psychiatrist Frank Ervin and neurosurgeon Vernon Mark.[24] Their suggestion that disease of the limbic system might underlie socially significant violent behavior, coupled with the implicit notion that surgical methods might be appropriate for the management of criminal violence, contributed to a heated public controversy concerning the surgery of violence and to the more general application of psychosurgical methods for control of socially deviant behavior.

The issues raised by the Ervin-Mark thesis are of considerable importance and subtlety. The core of their argument is that violent behavior, while influenced by social and psychological factors, is intrinsically an expression of brain activity, and that dysfunction of portions of the limbic system can condition, or in some cases actually generate, "senseless" violence. While the major premise in this argument is unexceptionable, since all behavior derives from brain activity, the idea that violence is specifically attributable to limbic system abnormality must be examined carefully. There is a considerable but not fully conclusive body of evidence which implicates the limbic system, especially the amygdala, in violent behavior. The main basis for presumption of an association between limbic system dysfunction and violence is, of course, the animal-derived observations that stimulation of the amygdala or posterior hypothalamus can trigger aggressive behavior, and that, conversely, lesions in these regions can produce a taming effect. In man, it has been asserted by some, most notably the British neurosurgeon Falconer along with Ervin and Mark, that epilepsy involving the temporal lobes may commonly be associated with aggressive and violent behavior. Mark and his colleagues have observed one case in which violent behavior was associated with grossly abnormal electrical activity recorded from the region of the amygdala. There is also statistical evidence for an increase in EEG abnormalities in prisoners incarcerated for violent crimes.[24] But looking at the other side of the coin, some patients with implanted electrodes have failed to show any evidence of abnormal discharge associated with episodes of violence, and it is clear that most temporal lobe epileptics are not violent. While some individuals have a strong propensity for violent behavior, it is not at all evident that these persons are suffering from disease of the limbic system.

Despite the fact that the association between temporal lobe epilepsy and violent behavior may be adventitious, the Boston group has limited their use of amygdalotomy to patients with coexisting temporal lobe epilepsy and behavioral disorder.[25] Although this limitation has the practical value of limiting the indiscriminate use of an unproven and possibly objectionable surgical treatment of violent individuals this decision serves to confound a number of critical issues in the surgical treatment of both epilepsy and violence.

It should be noted that the standard surgical treatment of temporal lobe epilepsy, the anterior temporal lobectomy, is performed only when seizures cannot be controlled by anticonvulsant drug treatment. This surgery is not performed for purely psychological indications, nor is it necessarily effective in ameliorating personality disorders when these coexist with the epilepsy. Amygdalotomy and other stereotaxic lesions within the temporal lobes have been tried in temporal lobe epilepsy, particularly when the disease is bilateral and lobectomy is therefore contraindicated. However, these stereotaxic procedures have not as yet been shown to be an effective therapeutic approach to these forms of epilepsy.

Amygdalotomy, when performed on patients suffering from epilepsy who also manifest aggressive behavior, should not be considered merely as treatment of epilepsy. Because of its behavioral effects, it must also be viewed as psychosurgery. It would seem wise to consider not only the nature of the therapeutic intent, but also the potential psychological changes which may be incurred as the result of surgery as proper criteria for identifying a procedure as psychosurgery. (The problem of definition is discussed at length by Joel Meister in Chapter 6.) This practice would direct greater attention to the need for careful assessment of psychological risks even when surgery is performed for what are primarily "neurological" conditions. Of particular relevance is the use of frontal lobotomy in the treatment of intractable pain. While this procedure is not psychosurgery in the classical sense, since the person is not mentally ill, Sweet has pointed out[45] that the psychological deficits in his patients lobotomized for pain were substantially greater than in psychiatric patients. It is likely that the deficiencies he noted in the patients without severe mental disorders were obscured by the psychopathology of the psychiatric patients.

The rationale for accepting surgical intervention in the abnormal brain more readily than in the supposedly normal one needs careful consideration. In a sense, all "abnormal" behavior represents an "abnormality" of brain function. Present knowledge concerning brain mechanisms is insufficient, however, to permit us to identify unequivocally particular electrophysiologic or chemical deviation as clearly pathological. There is a further difficulty in that the *causal* significance of a particular pathologic finding, even if the criteria of abnormality could be agreed upon, would remain moot, in the absence of a specific etiology. In any event, human brain processes are not readily monitored by present clinical techniques, so the detection of biological brain dysfunction which might underlie a given behavioral disorder is rarely possible at this time. The presence of organic brain pathology in epilepsy or mental retardation merely provides an excuse to allow the infliction of further structural damage to the brain in trying to eliminate the objectionable behavior.

On the face of it, there seems to be no fundamental reason to proscribe surgical treatment of abnormal behavior in patients with "normal" brains while permitting patients with abnormal brains to be subjected to lesioning. Why should not the severity of the behavior disorder itself be the criterion? This, of course, is the argument for psychosurgery in the treatment of severe psychopathology. The presence of brain pathology is not a consideration in performance of frontal lobotomy. The speciousness of justifying functional brain surgery (i.e., surgery which does not remove specifically pathological tissue) by the presence of some identifiable brain abnormality must be recognized by both sides of the psychosurgery controversy. Those opposed to psychosurgery may soon find themselves outflanked by increasingly sophisticated techniques for identification of brain pathology. Indeed, it is virtually certain that a "mentalistic" definition of psychosurgery will have increasingly little meaning as knowledge of brain physiology increases. In the long run it will be necessary to face up to the implications of increasing knowledge of the physical basis of mental activity. While there may be some temporary justification for limiting drastic forms of physical brain manipulation to patients with proven brain pathology, it has to be recognized that this evades the issue concerning definition of criteria regarding the acceptable limits of brain manipulation to accomplish behavioral change.

Although limbic system surgery has to date been almost exclusively limited to patients with brain damage diagnosed in a medical setting, the most explosive public issues are raised by its potential application to individuals whose behavior has been identified as criminal, whether or not they can be diagnosed as suffering from some aberration of brain function. Questions arising from this possibility are extraordinarily complex, involving relations among criminality, psychopathology, and brain dysfunction. An additional problem is posed by the circumstance that a preponderance of persons imprisoned for criminal acts, as well as those hospitalized for serious psychopathology, are drawn from the lower social and economic strata of society—a situation which in the United States possesses racial as well as class implications. It is important in considering the issues surrounding psychosurgical management of violence to distinguish grossly pathological behavior, as manifested by multiple murders and sexual assaults, from impulsive acts of violence, often occurring under the influence of alcohol, which constitute by far the major incidence of violent behavior. One must also exclude the political dissident, no matter how violent, as well as the uncooperative and resistive prisoner who represents a major current concern of penal authorities in the context of "violent" behavior. Any confusion of the psychopathology of mass murderers and sexual molesters with the behavior of ghetto rioters or prison malcontents must be dispelled—thereby avoiding a blurring of categories which many on both sides of the current controversy seem willing to tolerate and even to foster.

One pressing concern regarding medical and penal policy must be with persons who can be universally recognized as criminally insane, generally after the perpetration of extraordinarily deviant acts which, by their very nature, imply the presence of mental disorder. Most of these individuals are involved in multiple murders or sexual assaults, or both. Since there is no uniform policy of dealing with such offenders, some will be found in prisons and others in mental institutions. The few efforts which have been made to study these individuals from a sophisticated psychiatric and medical viewpoint identify a diverse group of severely disturbed personalities, with only occasional evidence of associated brain dysfunction. Identifiable biological factors are believed to be of minor significance in most of these individuals, although comprehensive neurological studies have rarely been performed. We do not understand the reasons for the grossly deviant behavior of these individuals, and we are unable to predict that a given person will perpetrate a grave offense (although there are certain early personality features which would lead to a suspicion of serious psychopathology). It is equally unclear as to what should be done with these people once they have acted and been apprehended. There have been a variety of proposals for the biological treatment of these individuals, especially the sexual offenders. Regardless of what "treatments" are employed, whether castration, the use of drugs suppressing the male sex hormone, or hypothalamic surgery, there is serious question as to their effectiveness in "curing" socially dangerous personality disorders.

As previously pointed out, the effects of hypothalamic lesions on basic biologic drives and emotional behavior are both influenced by environmental circumstances and subject to recovery after the passage of time. A good deal of the clinical evidence on the effects of therapeutic brain lesions, whether inflicted for neurological or psychiatric indications, suggests that favorable effects may be temporary, with improvement over a period of months to years followed by recurrence of the original symptoms. It may be important to distinguish the effects of a procedure such as frontal lobotomy, which can produce lasting therapeutic effects by relieving a disruptive emotional state, thereby allowing reintegration of the personality from the possibly temporary suppression by psychosurgery of impulsive drive-related behavior. It seems unwise to suggest that submission to a surgical procedure could provide the basis for release from custody. The legal issues raised here are as complex as the medical ones and are closely examined by Harold Edgar in Chapter 5 and by Ronald Gass in Chapter 3.

It seems difficult under present circumstances to justify the lesioning of drive-related brain regions in man. Certainly better evidence, both as to the lasting effectiveness of such procedures in suppressing abnormal drive-related behavior as well as to the lack of untoward effects, constitutes a minimum requirement. It may well be a myth to suppose that society can do anything other than provide a reasonably humane segregation of persons suffering from severely deviant expressions of drives. If nothing else, the controversy surrounding the surgery of violence has served to focus the attention both of the public and of the biomedical community onto the need for a deeper understanding of the problems posed by efforts to place deviant behavior and its modification within the medical context. While we seem reconciled to the use of neuroactive drugs to treat or modify almost anything unpleasant, the notion of a direct surgical assault upon the brain, as opposed to a more covert pharmacologic one, gives most of us pause.

Electrical and Chemical Stimulation of the Brain

The source of the concerns elicited by psychosurgery contrasts strikingly with those associated with the proposed clinical applications of brain stimulation. In the first instance it is the irreversibility and inherently unpredictable effects which are the source of criticism, whereas in the latter it is the very flexibility and precision of the techniques which are cause for concern. Before examining this seeming paradox, it is necessary to review briefly some of the scientific information on stimulation of the brain by electricity or neuroactive chemicals.

The natural counterparts of electrical brain stimulation are the epileptic disorders, in which nerve cells manifest an unusual tendency to discharge in massive synchronous bursts which disrupt the normal orchestration of neural processes. These discharges may be clinically manifested either as an arrest of ongoing behavior, or more dramatically as "seizures" in which consciousness is lost, with or without gross motor convulsions. These "generalized seizures" represent a virtually total involvement of the nervous system in the abnormal discharge. But often, due to a local scar or other brain damage, the discharge may arise from a small area, typically in the cortex or in limbic system structures within the temporal lobe (the amygdala and hippocampus). The clinical manifestations of these "focal" seizures permitted clinicians of the nineteenth century, such as J. Hughlings Jackson, to infer the functional characteristics of the brain regions within which the seizures originated, complementing the observations of lesion effects.

In the experimental arena, a major advance in the analysis of brain function was accomplished in 1870 by Fritsch and Hitzig,[10] who applied electrical current to the cortex of dogs and elicited movements of the extremities not unlike those produced by focal epileptic seizures involving the same cortical region. A series of studies in experimental animals was carried out during the succeeding decades. These studies mapped in detail the motor areas of the brain. However, they shed little light on the cortical areas concerned with sensory functions, since the animals could only indirectly indicate the occurrence of a sensory experience by a behavioral response.

Shortly after Fritsch and Hitzig's experimental demonstration of cortical response to electrical stimulation, a Cincinnati surgeon, Roberts Bartholow, grasped an opportunity to confirm their observations in a human subject. Thrusting a stimulating probe through a cancerous opening in the skull of a maidservant, he achieved the first modification of human behavior by electrical brain stimulation, as well as inducing a series of convulsions which resulted in her death. History fails to record the fate of the surgeon, although it is noted that he was forced to leave town after publication of his bold experiment.

Notwithstanding this disastrous occurrence, stimulation of the human brain was being carried out at the turn of the century during operations for various kinds of brain pathology. At this time the specialty of neurosurgery was born. The pioneers of neurosurgery, such as Sir Victor Horsley, who was the first surgeon to operate extensively on the human brain for the removal of tumors, were often prominent brain scientists. Horsley was a leading student of electrical brain stimulation, having devoted his early work to the detailed mapping of the cortex of primates. Thus it was that neurosurgery developed within an atmosphere of intense scientific interest in all aspects of brain function, in which activities the surgeons were often leading figures.

Human cortical stimulation under local anesthesia, which permitted the patient to report his subjective experiences, was carried out by German neurologist and surgeon Otfrid Foerster, and later by Wilder Penfield and his colleagues at the Montreal Neurological Institute during surgery for the removal of cortical scars and other localized brain lesions.[32] These workers ultimately obtained a detailed functional map of the human cortex which has subsequently provided a guide for the removal of pathological cortical tissue while producing the least possible damage to critical sensorimotor and language processes. This knowledge has benefited untold numbers of patients undergoing brain surgery, although it was obtained primarily to advance understanding of fundamental brain mechanisms. Both Foerster and Penfield regarded their therapeutic surgery as an unparalleled opportunity to gain this knowledge, and they expected their patients to participate in these experiments as part of the price they paid for their treatment. While the risks incurred by the patients were minimal due to the care exercised in these studies, current restrictions on clinical experimentation might well have precluded these critical observations.

At the same time that the surface of the human brain was being mapped by the neurosurgeons, other brain scientists were beginning to explore deep brain regions in experimental animals with the stimulating probe. This work complemented the ablations of deep structures which had demonstrated the role of the hypothalamus and structures within the limbic system in emotional behavior. Ranson[33] and Hess[16] both showed that hypothalamic stimulation could induce behavior in cats which appeared characteristic of rage (this was similar to the results obtained by Bard[1] by disconnecting the higher brain centers from the hypothalamus). Later work has defined in greater detail the neural structures associated with aggressive behavior in animals. The animal work has delineated a system involving portions of the hypothalamus and amygdala in aggressive behavior—with stimulation inducing attack and lesions producing tameness. This misleadingly simple formulation has led to the clinical application of amygdalotomy and hypothalamotomy in managing violent behavior in man. However, it is not yet possible to specify, even in the species most carefully studied, the full behavioral ramifications of manipulation of limbic system structures. An important outgrowth of these studies has been the growing recognition of the complexity of "aggression" as a behavior and the extreme difficulty in extra-polating studies in one animal species to another—particularly to man. The significance of this caveat has yet to be fully appreciated by those who have used animal observations to justify efforts to suppress human violence through the use of brain lesions.

Experimental brain stimulation has disclosed effects of even greater significance for the experimental control of behavior. Delgado, Roberts, and Miller[7] showed that electrical stimulation of certain deep brain regions could be employed as a "negative reinforcement" in experimental conditioning. At almost the same time James Olds and Peter Milner[30] discovered the phenomenon of "self-stimulation." They found that an animal would repeatedly press a bar to deliver an electrical stimulus to his brain when the electrode was placed at specific sites within and near the hypothalamus. These experiments showed that an animal's behavior could be either rewarded or punished by delivering an electric shock to the appropriate brain region. Through pairing of reward or punishment with specific behaviors, the animal's behavior could be "shaped" to the will of the experimenter, according to well-known principles of operant conditioning.

It was speculated that the positive and negative reinforcing effects of intracranial stimulation were associated with "pleasura-ble" or "painful" experiences, but these suppositions could only be confirmed by stimulation of these deep brain regions in man. Only a few such observations have been made, but these have made it clear that human patients may experience both pleasura-ble as well as unpleasant feelings when stimulated at points within the limbic system. Psychiatrist Robert Heath[14] has even demon-strated self-stimulation behavior in a human schizophrenic patient whose brain was implanted with deep stimulating electrodes to explore the therapeutic possibilities of electrical stimulation in sites thought to be involved in producing the psychotic behavior. It appears that intracranial stimulation can be as potent a reinforcer of behavior in man as it is in experimental animals—a sobering thought, considering that a rat will self-stimulate to the point of collapse in preference to eating and drinking.

To sum up our present empirical knowledge of the effects of ESB gained from the study of man and experimental animals, we can identify three major categories of behavioral and physiologic effect:

1. Modification of affective mechanisms to produce changes in feelings and mood, as well as to serve as either positive or negative reinforcers of behavior. The effective sites are primarily within the limbic system.

2. Activation of sensory and motor regions of the brain to produce elementary or complex experiences or movements. The active areas include the primary and secondary cortical representations as well as subcortical regions involved in sensory functions or in the programming of movement.

3. Suppression or inhibition of behavior and/or experience. These effects, which may be associated with stimulation of many brain regions, may either reflect a disruption of ongoing brain mechanisms by the electrical stimulus or, in some instances, the activation of physiologic mechanisms of inhibition.

Each of these ESB effects has formed the basis for possible therapeutic applications. Before considering these potential clinical uses, a brief mention must be made of chemical brain stimulation. In contrast to electrical stimuli, which influence nerve cells in a relatively indiscriminate fashion, specific chemical agents can selectively activate or inhibit the activity of nerve cells according to their specific sensitivities. In recent years our understanding of the chemical basis for neural excitation and inhibition and of the specific actions of drugs on the nervous system has vastly increased. As ordinarily administered, neuro-active drugs exert their effects upon all nerve cells which are sensitive to the particular substance. However, by administering small amounts of a drug, using a tiny pipette, the drug effects can be limited to a relatively circumscribed group of nerve cells, thus eliciting a rather precise physiologic response. These changes in neural activity may in turn be associated with specific behavioral effects.

The local application of neuroactive chemicals is at present a strictly investigative technique. The hypothesis that biochemical abnormalities, perhaps limited to certain brain regions, underlie some forms of mental illness raises the possibility that local application of specific chemicals might counteract these abnormalities. Even if this approach never becomes a practical therapeutic method, it might well form a critical part of the research necessary to identify conclusively the association between biochemical and behavioral disorders.

Perhaps because the removal or destruction of tissue is the classical therapeutic activity of surgeons, the development of therapeutic innovations in neurosurgery has, until quite recently, been limited almost exclusively to the development and refinement of methods for eradicating brain abnormalities either by removal of pathologic tissue, as in the surgical treatment of epilepsy, or by the presumptive disruption of pathophysiologic processes, as in psychosurgery. Brain stimulation has been used mainly for diagnostic and investigative purposes. In recent years, however, the therapeutic potential for brain stimulation, either electrical or chemical, has been increasingly recognized as providing an alternative to destructive procedures,[7,44] as in the treatment of epilepsy, or as a unique therapeutic innovation in the area of sensory and motor prosthesis. Some proposals, namely the use of complex patterned stimulation of the visual cortex to provide an artificial sensory input for the blind;[40] stimulation of the cerebellum to suppress epileptic seizures[12] or to reduce spasticity of the limbs after stroke; and certain attempts to modify behavior and mood in psychiatric patients[14] have all received a limited clinical trial by a tiny group of bold innovators. These activities have been controversial, due to scientific criticism of their conceptual and empirical basis as well as to broader concerns regarding the ethical aspects of the experimentation itself and the social implications of a successful outcome.

All of these factors have inhibited research into the use of human brain stimulation for therapeutic purposes. The various applications of intracranial stimulation must be distinguished from one another and evaluated on their individual merits rather than lumped together in the sort of pejorative categorization enjoyed by psychosurgery. Although all procedures involving brain manipulation deserve careful monitoring and evaluation, the problems posed by implementation of a visual prosthesis are of a different

59

nature from those involved in behavior modification using intracranial stimulation as a reinforcer.

Our present concerns are specifically related to the use of brain stimulation as a means of modifying psychological function. Techniques are now available, employing stereotaxic methods of placement, to deliver electrical or chemical stimulation to virtually any desired site within the human brain while producing minimal damage to the tissues through which the probes are passed. By stimulating various sites within the limbic system, it is possible to accomplish mood changes which may last for hours after brief electrical stimulation[8] or, after identifying "rewarding" or "punishing" sites, to accomplish behavioral changes through positive or negative reinforcement. As yet, neither of these effects has been exploited clinically in more than a handful of cases.

Indeed, only in one patient described by Heath[15] has the conditional association of intracranial stimulation with environmental manipulation been employed deliberately to alter a major aspect of the personality. In this case, an apparently successful effort was made to change the sexual preference of a homosexual male by pairing intracranial stimulation which produced erotic feelings with visual presentation of heterosexual activity. While this pornographic material initially produced revulsion, after brain stimulation the patient became sexually aroused and eventually achieved a full expression of heterosexual activity. Whatever the justification for this therapeutic exercise, it apparently demonstrated the potency of intracranial stimulation in modifying a type of behavior notably resistant to modification by usual psychotherapeutic methods.

Although there is little doubt of the potency of brain stimulation as a reinforcer when skillfully employed, there are inherent limitations in the potential scope of application to behavior modification. The most obvious is the requirement for surgical implantation of stimulating electrodes. This must be done by neurosurgeons skilled in stereotaxic techniques, and the practice is subject to controls which exist within the medical framework. At present these are largely self-imposed through a general recognition of the experimental nature of therapeutic brain stimulation. Thus we have the paradoxical situation that brain stimulation done prior to destructive surgery is not experimental, whereas the same procedure as a therapy is almost universally viewed as such. At this time, therefore, there is a circumscribed arena within which abuses might occur. The risks are mainly those common to psychosurgery, namely the lack of adequate scientific, clinical, and ethical standards by which applications of the procedure may be assessed. A far greater problem would exist if, through some unexpected but not impossible discovery, it became possible to deliver focal brain stimulation through the intact skull. Under these circumstances, given man's proven propensity to manipulate his own brain using drugs and novel techniques, such as biofeedback, a serious risk of uncontrolled self-stimulation could arise.

The use of intracranial reinforcement for behavior modification is also constrained by the need for sophisticated environmental manipulation. The control of reinforcement contingencies for behavioral shaping requires skills which are not often found in medical settings. In striking contrast to psychosurgery, wherein placement of the lesion constitutes the treatment, the therapeutic application of brain stimulation requires a continuing linkage between stimulation and monitoring of the patient's behavior. These exacting technical demands insure that the use of brain stimulation for behavior modification will never be a feasible method for large-scale clinical use, but will be limited in application to a small group of severe behavior disorders.

The requirement for consistent pairing of behavior with reinforcement also means that there are practical limits to the complexity of behavior which can be reliably influenced by operant techniques. The most impressive demonstrations of the potency of operant conditioning involve behaviors which can be precisely specified and are thus rather stereotyped. This restriction, which is a technical one, is nevertheless a significant constraint upon practical application of operant methods to the shaping of complex behaviors. Since operant conditioning generally requires a sharp focus upon a specific and manageable operant, it has proven difficult in practice to achieve "generalization." The shaping of a specific behavior may not lead to changes in related aspects of behavior. For this reason the specificity of operant techniques may represent a serious limitation on their therapeutic potential.

It is neither possible nor desirable to program all aspects of behavior to specific reinforcement contingencies. One would like to set a particular example and have this used as a model for the self-determination of a whole pattern of behavior. "As the twig is bent, so is the tree inclined" is a cardinal precept of education which contrasts strikingly with the circumscribed effects of the typical operant training. It is true that this limitation may also be technical in nature, due to the difficulty in selecting operant paradigms which influence more general classes of behavior. We are, however, very poor at defining the specific conditions which foster adaptive behavior.

The main problem in the development of optimal behavior patterns is not in achieving effective reinforcement, important as this may be, but in defining the behavior to be expressed. It may not be within our power so to define the limits of human activity, nor would it necessarily be desirable were it possible. The controversy surrounding the Skinnerian vision of a Utopian society exemplifies this problem.[39] Nevertheless, we have in operant conditioning a potent technique for affecting specific behaviors such as fighting, bedwetting, and autistic withdrawal. Whether behavioral disorders ever pose threats profound enough to the individual's well-being or to social welfare as to be an appropriate target for operant retraining employing intracranial reinforcement is a question which is probably not within our power at *this* time to answer for *all* time. It seems unlikely, however, that intracranial reinforcement could achieve general medical recognition as an acceptable form of therapy, except under the most unusual circumstances. These might be found in certain severely disabling behavioral disorders which are resistant to all other forms of treatment.

Another manner in which intracranial stimulation might be employed in psychiatric treatment utilizes the capacity of electrical stimulation of points within the limbic system to induce lasting changes in mood. Such effects have been reported both by Ervin and Mark[8,24] and by Heath.[14,15] It has been possible to modify a patient's basically aggressive and hostile attitude to one of ease and friendliness, a change not unlike that which had been reported to occur in monkeys after stimulation of certain intracranial sites. Such emotional modifications, especially feelings of well-being, could have a favorable effect upon states of chronic pain and anxiety which now might be treated by destructive surgery. Again, the frankly experimental nature of this application and the need for intracranial intrusion pose substantial difficulties for its implementation. Exploration of this therapeutic possibility is probably no more likely to be favored in the present climate of public opinion than the use of brain stimulation as a reinforcer in behavior modification.

Decisions concerning the further development of intracranial stimulation for behavior modification will turn on the resolution of the questions raised concerning all potent methodologies of behavior control. How are the goals of behavior change to be defined—and by whom? It will be necessary for the discipline of psychopathology to define with greater precision the means for identifying mental illness. More will also need to be known concerning the underlying brain mechanisms of deviant behaviors which might be considered sufficiently severe to warrant intra-cranial intervention. There is a critical need for a more adequate scientific definition of mental illness, so as to permit rational decisions concerning appropriate forms of therapy.

Physical Manipulation of the Brain—Prospectus

Many well-informed persons, even those deeply involved in the scientific study of brain and behavior, harbor grave concerns regarding approaches to the modification of human behavior employing direct manipulation of the brain. These concerns extend to the incautious and increasingly widespread use of psychoactive drugs, whether medically prescribed or self-administered. In a normal person there seems to be little, if anything, to be gained from tampering with the neural apparatus which millennia of evolutionary competition have brought to a high level of adaptive capacity. Indeed, the current extensive use of pharmacologic agents, whether for the purposes of blunting or "expanding" consciousness, appears to represent more a failure of adaptation to social stress than a means for improving man's condition in nature.

While acknowledging this personal bias toward "natural law," it must be admitted that through empirical science man has achieved a significant capacity to ameliorate some of the biological and psychological deviations which we call illnesses. To the extent that the therapies which have ensued from this quest are indeed effective and do not pose unacceptable risks for the patient, they find general acceptance within the medical profession and by society at large. Both of these groups expect, however, a strict adherence to the Hippocratic doctrine that the physician's first duty is to do no harm to his patient. Unfortunately, whenever knowledge is less than complete concerning efficacy and safety of a contemplated therapy, there arises a risk which is calculable only in a statistical sense. The physician is placed in a bind by the countervailing knowledge that the disease itself may carry a prognosis of sufficient gravity to threaten the future well-being or even the life of his patient. He must always weigh these uncertain factors, which are often complex and frequently ill-defined in quantitative terms, in arriving at a therapeutic decision. Such decisions are often called the "art" of medicine, since they involve intangible judgments concerning the nature of the patient's interests, often influenced by the physician's own values. Therapeutic decisions in the treatment of mental illness are among the most difficult in medicine, and are further conditioned by the knowledge that the available treatments are often ineffective. It is within this difficult therapeutic context that the validity of psychosurgery as well as newer, virtually untried techniques for physical brain manipulation must be assessed.

To complicate this issue further, the field of psychopathology lacks the "objective" diagnostic criteria of general medicine. Although pain may bring the ulcer patient to the physician, he need not rely merely on the patient's symptoms to establish the diagnosis. Not only can an ulcer be *seen* by the radiologist, but its existence can also be verified beyond doubt by the pathologist's examination of surgically removed tissue. In contrast, psychopathology exists only as syndromes of behavioral and experiential deviation. This results in diagnostic uncertainties which pose serious problems for selection and assessment of therapy. What constitutes a rational approach to the treatment of behavioral disturbances? How are decisions to apply a given treatment to be made? How is the effectiveness of treatment to be judged? By whose standards of behavior?

The seriousness of this diagnostic uncertainty has been underscored by comparisons of severe psychopathology made by psychiatrists in the United Kingdom and the United States.[5] The American psychiatrists diagnosed schizophrenia more frequently than their British counterparts, who favored the diagnosis of affective psychosis. This discrepancy seriously confounds comparisons between the two countries of treatment effectiveness in schizophrenia. This could account for the fact that the early American studies of frontal lobotomy, which included large numbers of schizophrenics, reported favorable responses in a substantial proportion of these patients. More recent data, from Britain, where psychosurgery is now performed more widely than in the U.S., has shown lobotomy to be relatively ineffective in schizophrenia, but efficacious in affective disorders.

The difficulties and discrepancies in psychiatric diagnosis create a fertile soil for claims that mental illness is a myth imposed upon the hapless and socially oppressed. If true, this assertion would challenge the validity of all biological approaches to the treatment of mental illness. Although the rational basis for the use of somatic therapies (drugs, insulin and electroconvulsive therapies, and psychosurgery) in mental illness is weak, the physician does believe that he is treating an illness rather than merely fostering or imposing arbitrary social norms. Since even "normal" behavior represents a synthesis of biological potentialities and environmental conditions, there is always an inextricable mix of social and biological factors in the genesis and expression of mental illness, and it is always a social decision as to how to regard behavioral deviation. Some societies may worship the deviant, others may condemn him. Such circumstances do not, however, vitiate the contribution of biological factors to mental disorders.

65

From the standpoint of biological therapies two intrinsically different rationales can be definied.

1.   A specific biological aberration may be identified and then corrected or ameliorated by an appropriate biochemical, pharmacologic, or physiologic manipulation. The behavioral manifestations caused by the disorder may thus be improved, or at least freed from the noxious effects of the underlying biologic disturbance. Such a condition is exemplified by the psychosis due to deficiency of vitamin B12, incurred by the absence of a substance required to permit its absorption into the body from food in the gut. The patient is cured by injection of the vitamin. Biological disorders, possibly due to an enzyme lack associated with a genetic change, are widely regarded as a likely basis for other psychoses, including schizophrenia and severe affective disorders.

2.   The treatment is directed against an identified behavioral aberration or constellation of symptoms without knowledge of the underlying pathogenic mechanisms. These symptomatic approaches must almost always be empirical, rather than based upon a rational attack upon etiology or pathophysiology. Most somatic treatment in psychiatry falls under this rubric.

It is probable that the very nature of the mechanisms which underlie behavior precludes application of the biologic model of causality to most manifestations of psychopathology. Even in the presence of a specific brain disturbance, removal of the pathologic influence may well leave the patient a psychological cripple, still prey to the patterns of maladaptive behavior learned during the morbid period. Since in most instances we do not have knowledge of the mechanisms underlying psychopathology, empirical therapies may for some time be the main avenue open to psychiatrists. The issues then become: When is treatment indicated? What are the goals of treatment? What therapies are most likely to be effective in gaining the desired outcome without damaging the integrity of the patient?

The lack of an identifiable pathological basis for the definition of mental disorders leaves the area open to definitions biased in accordance with dominant social concepts. This is one reason for maintaining a high degree of professional protection from capricious public and political influence or regulation. Whenever social factors unduly influence the definition and treatment of mental illness, these should be vigorously exposed and combated, but always on the basis of specific and valid complaints rather than as blanket condemnation of psychiatric diagnoses and therapies. At this time the controversy regarding psychosurgery and other somatic therapies, including drugs, has taken on the character of an ideological struggle in which consideration of the facts concerning the nature of mental illness and the actual effects of therapy have played a rather insignificant part. There is a great need, in moving toward policy decisions in this area, for dispassionate consideration of psychopathology and the various therapeutic alternatives under optimal conditions of scientific evaluation, supported by an informed public.

Clinical investigation will play a large role in this endeavor. In the absence of a perfect therapeutic armamentarium, based upon full understanding of the mechanisms underlying the conditions being treated, there will always be a search for better methods of therapy. At some point therapeutic innovations must be put to a clinical trial to determine their worth and risk under actual conditions of practice. It is often possible to delay this test until a significant indication of relative risks and benefits can be derived from animal studies. But especially in the area of psychopathology, animal models are either imperfect or lacking, so that clinical experimentation is the only feasible course. Society has refined its respect for the integrity of the person since the days in which criminals were subject to vivisection. We now demand that procedures recognized as experimental be carried out only under optimal scientific conditions with the informed consent of the subject or a suitable proxy. Although these requirements have been widely recognized and accepted since promulgation of the Nuremberg Code, practical circumstances have significantly limited their force.

These limitations are especially important with respect to the development of therapeutic innovations involving physical brain manipulation. First of all, it is necessary to define what therapies are to be considered "experimental" and thus subject to the accepted scientific and ethical principles. Accidents of clinical practice play a large role. Surgical innovations have historically been individual contributions of creative surgeons rather than the product of elaborate scientific study. While they may have been based upon laboratory findings, the first application to a human patient has generally represented a bold decision by one man or a small group of therapists. Traditionally, these decisions have not been formally subject to peer review. Thus, as in the case of psychosurgery, many surgeons strongly dispute the contention that these procedures are experimental even though their effectiveness and safety have not been established by recognized methods of clinical evaluation. There is possibly a confusion here between the *technique* and the *outcome*. The surgeon views the practice of stereotaxic surgery as well-founded in experimental and clinical experience. However, it is not the technique per se which is experimental, but rather its application to the treatment of mental illness. The surgeon is rarely equipped by training to decide that psychosurgery is justified for a specific patient by the severity of psychopathology and lack of response to alternative therapies; nor is he able to evaluate adequately the preoperative and postoperative psychological status of the patient. Other critical factors, which include social pressures on the patient and his potential for a satisfactory life adjustment, are often beyond the assessment capabilities of surgical practitioners. The literature reveals much attention to technical factors, but little appreciation of the nature of the psychiatric and psychosocial conditions being "treated." Often the psychological and psychiatric evaluations have been performed either by the surgeon himself, or by personnel of questionable professional qualifications. In the face of these critical inadequacies in clinical evaluation, there is a clear need for psychosurgery, broadly defined, to be placed within the category of "experimental therapies" and thus subject to optimal conditions of scientific and ethical review.

Even if it were possible to develop a mechanism for adjudicating the experimental status of specific therapies, such as psychosurgery, the experimental label would not necessarily safeguard the patient or insure the progress of valid clinical experimentation and needed assessments of innovative therapies. Mere establishment of controls might inhibit research altogether in those institutions which establish strict scientific and ethical review procedures and relegate questionable activities to institutions controlled by those favoring a particular procedure. The development of "underground psychosurgery" might be fostered by the principled support of some practitioners as well as by economic considerations.

An alternative to this potentially unsavory and therapeutically reactionary approach would require encouragement and support of research to improve the definition, evaluation, and longitudinal analysis of mental illness under the circumstances of our contemporary society. The required clinical research facilities should provide for an intensive and sustained review of the status of any psychopathology deemed sufficiently severe and chronic as to warrant direct intervention into the brain. Such studies must be undertaken within the broader context of psychopathology and psychiatric treatment so that detailed assessments of the indications for specific treatments and of their effectiveness and safety can emerge. As pointed out in the 1950 Conference on Psychosurgery sponsored by the NIMH,[35] it is not realistic to carry out such studies in many existing psychiatric facilities, due to their grossly inadequate staffing patterns. It is essential for a valid therapeutic assessment not only that optimal therapy of all appropriate kinds be available to the patients under study, but that the patients be followed for prolonged periods during and after their treatment. The clinical and scientific requirements for such studies are substantial and expensive.

Nevertheless, a rational approach to improvement of methods of psychiatric diagnosis and treatment requires the establishment of adequate institutional research facilities for application and comparative evaluation of innovative therapeutic approaches, regardless of the difficulties this may entail. The long-range costs, both human and economic, of such a course would surely be less than the continued expenditure of therapeutic effort without adequate evidence of favorable overall effects.

In the meantime there is an urgent need to institute effective measures for safeguarding the individual patient against unwarranted or incompetent physical intervention upon his nervous system. Some of the steps which seem appropriate for accomplishing this end are outlined and discussed by Harold Edgar (Chapter

5) and Ronald Gass (Chapter 3). Of greatest importance for the continuing scientific and public discourse concerning the medical and social implications of techniques for physical manipulation of the brain will be a reevaluation of the human context in which such therapies are proposed—a reevaluation demanded by increasing knowledge of the physical basis of man's mental activities.

REFERENCES

1. Bard, P., and Mountcastle, V. B. "Some Forebrain Mechanisms Involved in Expression of Rage with Special Reference to Suppression of Angry Behavior." *Research Publications of the Association for Research in Nervous and Mental Disease* 27 (1948): 362-404.

2. Bianchi, L. "The Functions of the Frontal Lobes." *Brain* 18 (1895): 497-530.

3. Columbia-Greystone Associates. *Selective Partial Ablation of the Frontal Cortex*, edited by F. A. Mettler. New York: Hoeber, 1949.

4. Columbia-Greystone Associates (Second Group). *Psychosurgical Problems*, edited by F. A. Mettler. Philadelphia: Blakiston, 1952.

5. Cooper, J. E.; Kendell, R. E.; Gurland, B. J.; Sharpe, L.; Copeland, J. R. M.; and Simon, R. J. *Psychiatric Diagnosis in New York and London: A Comparative Study of Mental Hospital Admissions*. Maudsley Monograph #20. London: Oxford University Press, 1972.

6. Delgado, Jose M. R. *The Physical Control of the Mind*. New York: Harper & Row, 1969.

7. Delgado, Jose M. R.; Roberts, W. W.; and Miller, N. E. "Learning Motivated by Stimulation of the Brain. *American Journal of Physiology* 179 (1954): 587-593.

8. Ervin, F. R.; Mark, V. H.; and Stevens, J. "Behavioral and Affective Responses to Brain Stimulation." *Neurobiological Aspects of Psychopathology*, edited by J. Zubin and C. Stagass. pp. 54-65. New York: Grune & Stratton, 1969.

9. Freeman, W. "Frontal Lobotomy in Early Schizophrenia: Long Follow-Up in 415 Cases." In *Psychosurgery: Proceedings of the Second International Conference*, edited by E. Hitchcock; L. Laitinen; and K. Vaernet, p. 311-321. Springfield, Ill.: Charles C. Thomas, 1972.

10. Fritsch, G. and Hitzig, E. "Über die Elektrische Erregbankeit des Grosshirns." *Archiv fuer Anatomie, Physiologie und Wissenschaftliche Medicin* 37 (1870): 300-332.

11. Fulton, J. F. *Frontal Lobotomy and Affective Behavior. A Neurophysiological Analysis*. New York: Norton, 1951.

12. Cooper, I. S.; Amin, I.; and Gilman, S. "The Effect of Chronic Cerebellar Stimulation upon Epilepsy in Man." In *Transactions of the American Neurological Association*, edited by Samuel A. Trufant, New York: Springer Publishing Co., 1973, pp. 192-196.

13. Greenblatt, Milton and Solomin, H. C. *Frontal Lobes and Schizophrenia; Second Lobotomy Project of Boston Psychopathic Hospital*. New York: Springer, 1953.

14. Heath, R. G., ed. *The Role of Pleasure in Behavior*. New York: Hoeber-Harper & Row, 1964.

15. Heath, R. G. "Pleasure and Brain Activity in Man." *Journal of Nervous and Mental Diseases* 154 (1972): 3-18.

16. Hess, W. R. *The Functional Organization of the Diencephalon*. New York: Grune & Stratton, 1957.

17. Hitchcock, E.; Laitinen, L.; and Vaernet, K., eds. *Psychosurgery: Proceedings*

of the Second International Conference. Springfield, Ill.: Charles C. Thomas, 1972.

18. Jacobsen, C. F. "Influence of Motor and Premotor Area Lesions upon the Retention of Acquired Skilled Movements in Monkeys and Chimpanzees." *Research Publications of the Association for Research in Nervous and Mental Disease* 13(1934):225-247.

19. Klüver, H. and Bucy, P. C. "An Analysis of Certain Effects of Bilateral Temporal Lobectomy in the Rhesus Monkey with Special Reference to Psychic Blindness." *Journal of Psychology*. 5 (1938): 33-54.

20. Lashley, K. S. *Brain Mechanisms and Intelligence*. Chicago: University of Chicago Press, 1929.

21. Lewis, N. D.; Landis, C.; and King, H. E., eds. *Studies in Topectomy*. New York: Grune & Stratton, 1956.

22. McCleary, R. A. and Moore, R. Y. *Subcortical Mechanisms of Behavior*. New York: Basic Books, 1965.

23. McEwen, B. S.; Zigmond, R. E.; and Gerlach, J. L. "Sites of Steroid Binding and Action in the Brain." In *The Structure and Function of Nervous Tissue*, edited by G. H. Bourne, pp. 205-291. New York: Academic Press, 1972.

24. Mark, V. H. and Ervin, F. R. *Violence and the Brain*. New York: Harper & Row, 1970.

25. Mark, V. H. and Neville, R. "Social and Ethical Implications of Brain Surgery in Aggressive Epileptics." *Journal of the American Medical Association* 226(1973): 765-772.

26. Miller, A., ed. *Lobotomy: A Clinical Study*. Toronto: Ontario Department of Health, 1954.

27. Milner, Brenda. "Brain Mechanisms Suggested by Studies of Temporal Lobes". In *Brain Mechanisms Underlying Speech and Language*, edited by F. L. Darley, pp. 122-145. New York: Grune & Stratton, 1967.

28. Moniz, E. *Tentatives Opératoires Dans Le Traitement De Certaines Psychoses*. Paris: Masson, 1936.

29. Narabayashi, H. and Uno, M. "Long-range Results of Stereotaxic Amygdalotomy for Behavioral Disorder." *Confinia Neurologica* 27 (1966):168-171.

30. Olds, J. and Milner, P. "Positive Reinforcement Produced by Electrical Stimulation of Septal Area and Other Regions of Rat Brain." *Journal of Comparative and Physiological Psychology* 47 (1954):419-427.

31. Penfield, W. and Jasper, H. H. *Epilepsy and the Functional Anatomy of the Human Brain*. Boston: Little, Brown, 1954.

32. Penfield, W. and Rasmussen, T. *The Cerebral Cortex of Man*. New York: Macmillan, 1950.

33. Ranson, S. W. "Some Functions of the Hypothalamus." *Harvey Lectures* 32 (1937): 92-121.

34. Research Conference Group on Psychosurgery, 1951 "Criteria for the Selection of Psychotic Patients for Psychosurgery." *Proceedings of the First Research Conference on Psychosurgery (1949)*. F. A. Mettler, Chairman, N. Bigelow, Editor (Public Health Service Publication No. 16) Washington, D.C.: U.S. Government Printing Office.

35. Research Conference Group on Psychosurgery, 1952. "Evaluation of Change in Patients after Psychosurgery." *Proceedings of the Second Research Conference on Psychosurgery (1950)*. F. A. Mettler, Chairman, W. Overhosler, Editor (Public Health Service Publication No. 156). Washington, D.C.: U.S. Government Printing Office.

36. Research Conference Group on Psychosurgery, 1954. "Evaluation of Psychosurgery." *Proceedings of the Third Research Conference on Psychosurgery (1951)*. F. A. Mettler, Chairman, W. Overholser, Editor (Public Health Service Publication No. 221) Washington, D.C.: U.S. Government Printing Office.

37. Sano, Keiji. Personal Communication.

38. Scoville, W. B. and Milner, Brenda. "Loss of Recent Memory After Bilateral Hippocampal Lesions." *Journal of Neurology, Neurosurgery and Psychiatry* 20(1957): 11-21.

39. Skinner, B. F. *Walden Two*. New York: Macmillan, 1948.

40. Sterling, T. D.; Bering, E. A., Jr.; Pollack, S. V.; and Vaughan, H. G., Jr. *Visual Prosthesis—The Interdisciplinary Dialogue*. New York: Academic Press, 1971.

41. Teitelbaum, P. and Epstein, A. N. "The Lateral Hypothalamic Syndrome: Recovery of Feeding and Drinking After Lateral Hypothalamic Lesions." *Psychological Review* 69(1962):74-90.

42. Teuber, H. L. "The Riddle of Frontal Lobe Function in Man." In *The Frontal Granular Cortex and Behavior*, edited by J. M. Warren and K. Akert, pp. 410-477. New York: McGraw-Hill, 1964.

43. Tow, P. M. *Personality Changes Following Frontal Leucotomy*. London: Oxford University Press, 1955.

44. Vaughan, H. G., Jr. "Some Reflections on Stimulation of the Human Brain." In *Neurobiological Aspects of Psychopathology*, edited by J. Zubin and C. Shagass, pp. 66-77. New York: Grune & Stratton, 1969.

45. White, J. C., and Sweet, W. H. *Pain and the Neurosurgeon*. Springfield, Ill.: Charles C. Thomas, 1969.

3 / Kaimowitz v. Department of Mental Health: The Detroit Psychosurgery Case

IN MID-JANUARY 1973, two staff physicians at Detroit's prestigious Lafayette Clinic, a state-funded research facility, were preparing to initiate a study designed to compare the efficacy of two experimental treatment techniques—psychosurgery and drug intervention—for the control of aggressive behavior. Dr. Ernst Rodin, Chief of Neurology at Lafayette, and his colleague, Dr. J. S. Gottlieb, a psychiatrist and the director of the clinic, had scheduled a thirty-six-year-old mental patient for the implantation of depthelectrodes in order to detect and monitor electrical abnormalities in his brain's limbic system, the theorized controlling mechanism for rage reactions. Once an area of dysfunction had been located, it was to be destroyed by means of sterotactic surgery. No substantive objections had been raised concerning the research design's scientific validity or ethical propriety when it was reviewed and approved by several clinic and state legislature committees, and the coprincipal investigators maintained throughout the court proceedings that the subject's human and legal rights had been respected and scrupulously upheld.

Not everyone, however, believed that the serious ethical implications surrounding the Lafayette Clinic aggression project had been adequately resolved. On January 7 a front-page article appearing in the *Detroit Free Press* challenged the soundness of the research design and intimated that a number of procedural improprieties may have led to the illegal abrogation of the patient's civil rights.[1] Concurrently, a petition and complaint had been prepared and filed with the Wayne County Circuit Court by Gabe Kaimowitz, a senior staff attorney for the Michigan Medical Committee for Human Rights,[2] on behalf of its membership. The complaint included the following principal allegations:

1. Orders to show cause ... why John Doe [the pseudonym used to identify the first patient selected to participate in the Lafayette Clinic aggression project] and others are or will be involuntarily detained at Lafayette Clinic and why they [staff members at the clinic] should not be enjoined from performing psychosurgery or using chemotherapy on persons involuntarily confined in the state hospital system in order to study "treatment of uncontrollable aggression" or for any other similar purpose.
2. Writs of habeas corpus should issue releasing John Doe and others from involuntary confinement in state hospitals where they are not being treated, until such time as it is determined that they can be properly confined in appropriate institutions under existing state law.
3. Respondents should be enjoined from using state funds to conduct a study of the treatment of uncontrollable aggression or other behavior involving the use of means which have permanent effects, when the subjects of such study are not in positions to voluntarily consent to participation in such experimentation.[3]

The circuit court's three-judge panel was the first judiciary body in the United States to broach formally the medical, legal, and ethical implications of psychosurgery within the context of a total institution. Preliminary arguments were presented in early March 1973, at which time permission was granted the American

Orthopsychiatric Association to participate as amicus curiae. By March 15 the court ruled that the State Department of Mental Health's decision to terminate funding for the aggression project had not rendered the critical legal issues involved moot. Eight days later the court declared that the criminal sexual psychopath (CSP) statute under which John Doe had been committed was unconstitutional. Subsequently the judges framed the following two questions for declaratory judgment:

1. After failure of established therapies, may an adult or the legally appointed guardian, if the adult is involuntarily detained at a facility within the jurisdiction of the State Department of Mental Health, give legally adequate consent to an innovative or experimental surgical procedure on the brain, if there is demonstrable physical abnormality of the brain and the procedure is designed to ameliorate behavior which is either personally tormenting to the patient or so profoundly disruptive that the patient cannot safely live or live with others?

2. If the answer to the above question is yes, then is it legal in this state to undertake an innovative or experimental surgical procedure on the brain of an adult involuntarily detained at a facility within the jurisdiction of the State Department of Mental Health, if there is demonstrable physical abnormality of the brain and the procedure is designed to ameliorate behavior which is personally tormenting to the patient or so profoundly disruptive that the patient cannot safely live or live with others?[4]

Ironically, the State Department of Mental Health declined to initiate civil commitment proceedings against Doe on the grounds that he was not sufficiently "mentally ill" to warrant such action. And so, after 18 years of continuous confinement in state mental hospitals, Doe was freed in early April 1973.[5]

As a preface to the complete text of the court opinion in *Kaimowitz* v. *Department of Mental Health,* the following summary of events, based upon court testimony, interviews, and newspaper accounts, traces the origin and evolution of the Lafayette Clinic aggression project prior to legal action.

The initial impetus for the aggression project stemmed from the publication of an extremely provocative monograph entitled *Violence and the Brain,*[6] coauthored by Harvard physicians Vernon H. Mark, a neurosurgeon, and Frank R. Ervin, a psychiatrist. Their pioneering research has tentatively established correlations between electrical abnormalities within the brain's limbic system and outbursts of aggressive behavior, with particular emphasis on the role of the amygdala (an almond-shaped nucleus deep in the temporal cortex of the brain) in controlling rage reactions. *Violence and the Brain* details Mark and Ervin's experimental techniques and is embellished with several case histories of patients treated for aggressive behavior stemming directly from organic brain pathology, notably temporal lobe epilepsy. Briefly, the procedures they describe are as follows: (1) depthelectrography—an innovative diagnostic technique used to pinpoint areas of abnormal electrical activity deep within limbic system structure by means of stereotactically implanted electrodes;[7] (2) direct electrostimulation of certain portions of the brain via depthelectrodes in an effort to trigger episodes of aggressive behavior; (3) telemetric monitoring of spontaneous electrical impulses; and (4) remote stimulation of discrete brain structures as the subject interacts with others in a hospital ward setting, thereby enabling investigators to record and correlate neuroelectric responses with various cuing stimuli in the patient's environment.

Mark and Ervin's research leads them to postulate a link between abnormal electrical activity in various limbic system structures and aggressive behavior patterns. However, to establish such a correlation, an intermediate experiment is required. Since the Harvard group's studies concentrated on those individuals with a specific and verifiable form of pathology (i.e., temporal lobe epilepsy), it remains to be demonstrated whether or not people prone to episodic outbursts of uncontrollable rage but not suffering from a predisposing pathological condition also manifest abnormal electrical activity in their limbic system structures. One means of detecting such impulses would be to implant depthelectrodes in the apparently "normal" brains of subjects given to violent outbursts and then remotely monitor their neuroelectric activity when exposed to aggression-provoking stimuli. Unfortunately, the clinical criteria for distinguishing the "aggression-prone" individual from a "normal" subject remain so nebulous that ambiguous conclusions are practically unavoidable.

Drs. Rodin and Gottlieb read *Violence and the Brain* independently soon after its publication in 1970, and at Gottlieb's invitation the two of them met to discuss the merits of the Harvard group's research. They agreed that some of the techniques described in the monograph might be therapeutically advantageous for certain patients in the state hospital system who were suffering from uncontrollable sexual and aggressive impulses. Dr. Rodin proceeded to draft a five-page paper (see note 12), entitled "Proposal for the Study of the Treatment of Uncontrollable Aggression at the Lafayette Clinic," in which he outlines a comparative study of surgical versus medical treatment of mental patients subject to severe and uncontrollable outbursts of aggression. The stated goal of the project was restoration of the patient to "a useful life" within the community. The 12 patients of the surgical treatment series were to have depthelectrodes implanted in order to: (1) monitor neuroelectric activity; (2) stimulate various brain structures; and (3) detect focal points of electrical abnormality. If a specific area of the brain could be identified as the mechanism controlling aggressive responses definitive stereotactic surgery would be performed, resulting in the destruction of the area by either a block resection or electrocoagulation technique.

In conjunction with this first group, a second series of 12 mental patients, matched on the basis of sex, age, IQ, and similarity of episodic behavioral disturbances, would participate in the medical aspect of the study. Based upon the premise that the hormone testosterone is primarily responsible for aggressive behavior in males, cyproterone acetate (an antiandrogen agent) was to be administered to each subject to depress hormone production. This drug was developed by a West German pharmaceutical company and used extensively in Europe for the treatment of sexual offenders suffering from what some psychiatrists label as sex-related behavioral disturbances (e.g., pedophilia, homosexuality, excessive masturbation).

If either one of the treatment regimens succeeded in inducing a "calming effect" while improving stress tolerance to the point where the patient could safely be released, it was theorized that the subject would then be optimally receptive to state-sponsored rehabilitation programs. If one treatment modality proved more efficacious than the other, those in the less successful group were to be given that therapy.

In January 1971 Dr. Rodin was invited to present a paper before the Winter Conference of Brain Research symposium on aggression. Rodin's presentation dealt with some of the difficulties encephalographers face whenever they attempt to establish correlates between abnormal behavior and cerebral electrical activity, particularly in aggression-prone individuals. The paper clearly reflects his attitude toward the two treatment regimens included in the aggression project proposal. Rodin laments the fact that he is probably in the "woeful minority" when it comes to controlled experimental studies comparing the effects of castration against surgical procedures on the brain. He urges researchers to "get down to cold-blooded medical research dealing with individuals rather than masses" and thereby redirect our attention from global abstractions founded upon sociological considerations that lead us to spend billions of dollars on "ill-conceived do-good projects."[8] What is required, he admonishes, is an interdisciplinary team of researchers, representing the biological and behavioral sciences, which would concentrate upon the problem of aggressive-assaultive behavior to the temporary exclusion of all other concerns.

Accompanied by a $164,000 budget request, the aggression project proposal was submitted to the State Department of Mental Health for its consideration. It was subsequently approved for funding and incorporated as a "research" line item under the Lafayette Clinic budget which, in turn, was presented to the state legislature together with the entire 1972-1973 State Department of Mental Health request. Both the Michigan State Senate Appropriations Committee and the Subcommittee on Mental Health held hearings on health department expenditures, but neither group raised any specific objections to the aggression project proposal. Acting upon these committees' recommendations, the state legislature gave its "rubber stamp" approval just prior to the summer recess. The requested funds for the project were made available on July 1, 1972.

Once funding was assured, Dr. Rodin drafted a two-page series of guidelines entitled "Criteria for Inclusion in Aggression Project" to assist state hospital superintendents in making the proper referrals. Since the project was designed to treat only those patients suffering from severe episodes of uncontrollable aggressive behavior or sexual aggressive behavior, the few remaining criminal sexual psychopaths in state hospitals suddenly became the prime source for potential candidates.

Prior to 1968, Michigan had enforced a special criminal sexual psychopath statute enabling individuals facing serious charges relating to sexual assault to undergo psychological examinations to determine whether they qualify for detention under this law. If they met the CSP criteria, the court proceedings would be discontinued and the defendant could be admitted directly to a state mental hospital for treatment on an indeterminate, involuntary basis until a "cure" was effected. In 1968, however, the Michigan state legislature repealed the CSP statute, but a savings clause permitted continued detention of those already institutionalized. Since that time the State Department of Mental Health has been gradually releasing the 318 CSP patients committed to state hospitals. Despite the fact that the term "criminal sexual psychopath," which is legal rather than medical, does not appear in Dr. Rodin's criteria for inclusion, it became evident that almost any mental patient with a history of acted-out violence could fulfill the rather vague guidelines Rodin had established. During his testimony, Dr. Rodin did assert that only CSP patients in the state hospital system had been envisioned as potential candidates for the aggression project. In June 1972 a maximum of 50 criminal sexual psychopaths would have been available for the study, and by January 1973 all but 12 had been released.[9]

John Doe's candidacy for the project was first broached by Dr. E. G. Yudashkin, director of the State Department of Mental Health, during the course of a patient-staff meeting at Ionia State Hospital in May 1972.[10] At this time Yudashkin described the project to Doe, making it clear to him that he was being considered for release within six months to a year whether or not he decided to participate; however, it was also pointed out that awaiting discharge would clearly be more time consuming than successful completion of either of the two experimental treatment programs. Doe immediately declined to participate in the antiandrogen drug study but did express an interest in the surgical procedure. At his request he received three independent explanations of depthelectrography techniques from Dr. Yudashkin and two of the staff physicians at Ionia; however, Doe's testimony indicated that his conversations with the state hospital doctors left him with an extremely simplistic view of the proposed operation due to the physicians' own rudimentary knowledge of the procedures. Following later discussions with his parents and several fellow inmates, he decided to consent to the operation. Yudashkin, convinced of Doe's sincerity, referred him directly to Dr. Rodin as a potential candidate for depthelectrography and sterotactic surgery.

In the meantime, Rodin had arranged meetings with several prominent investigators in the area of psychosurgical control of aggressive behavior, including Drs. Vernon Mark and Jose Delgado. In a memorandum to Dr. Gottlieb on August 9, 1972, Rodin remarks that Mark and Ervin's book, *Violence and the Brain,* had misled them into believing that some of the patients treated by the Harvard researchers did not have demonstrable temporal lobe epilepsy. In light of this discovery, he affirms that "we cannot in good conscience suggest the operation of amygdalotomy to a patient who is aggressive but shows no evidence of temporal lobe disease."[11]

Because of the disappointing response to Dr. Rodin's original criteria for inclusion, an August 1972 meeting was arranged among Rodin, Yudashkin, and the neurosurgeon who was to perform the depthelectrode implant to discuss a possible revision. By verbal agreement they decided to rule out surgery on patients without verifiable organic brain dysfunctions, and to include those in the state hospital system who were retarded, epileptic, or self-mutilative. The potential research population was, in effect, expanded without altering the basic research design through the deletion of some of the more restrictive clauses included in the original inclusion criteria (e.g., exclusion of mental retardates). It was not until December 15 that Dr. Yudashkin issued a confidential memorandum to all state hospital superintendents embodying the aforementioned modifications.

Experimental projects at the Lafayette Clinic were subject to the review and approval of its eight-member Human and Animal Experimentation Committee, which examined all research protocols to assure that they protected adequately the rights and welfare of experimental subjects. Participation on this standing committee was limited to those staff members at Lafayette actively engaged in some facet of investigative and/or therapeutic medicine; hence, all of them were colleagues of Dr. Rodin. This panel would convene four times a year to consider a total of about 12 projects. By the end of August 1972 Dr. Rodin had submitted a copy of the aggression project protocol to this committee, but it was not until October 20 that it met to discuss the protocol. By this time Rodin had provided it with a revised version of the 1970 proposal and a draft of the informed consent form. After deliberating for less than an hour and a half over two independent research projects, the committee voted to approve Dr. Rodin's proposal. According to testimony, a number of questions concerning the research design were raised; however, the meeting's apparent brevity was accounted for by the fact that prior and less formal conversations (e.g., during lunch, in the hallways) between committee members and Drs. Gottlieb and Rodin had served as adequate occasions for discussion of the project.

The 1972 version of the aggression project protocol was virtually identical to the one drafted in 1970 except for the insertion of two additional paragraphs. They concern two special review committees which were to be established to oversee patient selection and protect them from unethical practices. A three-member "Medical Review Committee" was to consider the patients referred by Rodin on the basis of their medical history and background to "guard against operating on patients in whom the medical indication might be dubious."[12] Once this committee gave its approval, a three-member "Human Rights Review Committee" would then verify the adequacy of the informed consent form as well as interview the patient, if they wished, in order to "guard against infringement of the human rights of the patient."[13] When both committees concurred on the selection of a candidate, he would then be provided with the consent form and a detailed explanation of the proposed procedures by a member of the Department of Neurology from Lafayette Clinic. The patient and his family were to be given at least a week's time to consider the pros and cons of the treatment regimen prior to signing the consent form.

Since the Human and Animal Experimentation Committee was not charged with the responsibility of reviewing the scientific adequacy of experimental studies, the more technical aspects were considered at weekly research conferences. These colloquia purportedly were open to the entire Lafayette Clinic staff and interested members of the public. Here problems relating to research design could be reviewed by a fairly broad spectrum of the clinic's staff. The aggression project, however, was never presented at these meetings because it had been classified as a "pilot study," i.e., "a project differentiated from one which had a broader scope where it was more completely written up,"[14] and hence not subject to review at these conferences. Rodin's proposal was the first such pilot study to have been conducted at Lafayette Clinic in over two years.

In direct violation of the protocol established by the 1972 proposal revision described above, consent and review procedures were carried out as follows: On October 27 John Doe met with Dr. Rodin at Ionia State Hospital to discuss his participation in the aggression project. Following an hour-long conversation concerning his medical history, Doe reaffirmed his desire to participate in the surgical aspect of the study, and Dr. Rodin read him the informed consent form. Together they examined the document section by section to clarify the meaning and attendant risks of the surgical techniques it described. Following Rodin's departure, Doe was given permission to contact his parents, who arrived at Ionia that same evening. Prior to signing the consent form, the only explanation of the treatment procedures Doe's parents received came from their son. Doe believed erroneously that he and his parents were consenting *only* to the depthelectrography study and not the stereotactic psychosurgery procedure. They were all under the impression that their consent would be elicited a second time *after* the requisite diagnostic data had been collected. On November 6 Doe was transferred to Lafayette Clinic.

It was Dr. Rodin who finally determined who should sit on the two review committees he had established. According to testimony, Rodin had indicated to the chairman of the Human and

Animal Experimentation Committee that he believed a neurosurgeon, a neurologist, and a psychiatrist would be appropriate to sit on the Medical Review Committee, and in the end it was he who made the final selection. The three physicians on this panel never conferred, but did consider John Doe's candidacy individually, based solely on information forwarded by Dr. Rodin. It is important to note that this medical review was conducted *after* both Doe and his parents had signed the consent form.

Similarly, the three members of the Human Rights Review Committee (a clergyman, a law professor, and a representative of the community) were chosen by Rodin, who provided them with the following materials: the aggression project proposal (1972 revision); the original criteria for inclusion; background information on psychosurgery, with particular reference to the work of Mark and Ervin; and a social/medical profile of John Doe. This review panel viewed its primary function as the evaluation of the quality of the subject's informed consent, and not the determination of the research design's scientific adequacy. Hence, no committee at Lafayette had had an opportunity to challenge the veracity and soundness of the project's scientific foundation. Each member of the Human Rights Review Committee examined the proposal independently, conferring only once prior to the initiation of legal action in January 1973. In addition, the members of this panel were permitted to interview Doe individually; however, they never met to discuss the merits of Doe's case.

By the end of December 1972 all of the requisite committee reviews had been completed, and preparations were underway for the electrode implantation by early January, despite the fact that not a single patient, aside from John Doe, had been located to participate in either the surgical or medical treatment programs. According to Dr. Yudashkin's testimony, the aforementioned December 15 revision of the inclusion criteria[15] was actually intended to be a means of canvassing the state hospital system to determine whether a sufficiently large patient population existed which might benefit from participation in the aggression project. Theoretically, Doe should not have been allowed to participate in this study, since patients from any one of the modified categories could not be seriously considered for the project unless the entire proposal were resubmitted and approved by the state legislature. Even more surprising was Yudashkin's remark that the State Department of Mental Health reserved the right to restrict the number of subjects in the aggression project to any number less than 12 even though it did not have the authority to go beyond that limit. If this prerogative had been exercised, it clearly would have invalidated the study altogether, and the department would have been guilty of misrepresenting the scope and purpose of the project.

Sometime in late December 1972 Gabe Kaimowitz was contacted by a psychiatry resident from Lafayette Clinic who expressed his discomfort and concern over the surreptitious manner in which the aggression project was being conducted. Kaimowitz decided to investigate this report by contacting several other psychiatrists associated with the clinic who also were aware of Dr. Rodin's study and the impending depthelectrode implantation. After documenting their statements, Kaimowitz proceeded to draft a petition and complaint to enjoin the Lafayette Clinic and the State Department of Mental Health from continuing its support of the aggression project.

Concurrently, two staff reporters for the *Detroit Free Press* had been notified independently about the implant operation to be performed on John Doe, and soon after they arranged a luncheon appointment with Dr. Rodin to discuss the project. The January 7 edition of the *Free Press* carried the results of their interviews. A combination of adverse public reaction and revealing articles in nationally prominent newspapers prompted Dr. Yudashkin to announce that the State Department of Mental Health had terminated its support of the project by withholding all appropriated funding and withdrawing a pending budget renewal request in the amount of $172,995.

The above prologue to the court opinion (reprinted as Appendix) was intended to assist the reader in understanding the complex series of events underlying the implementation of the Lafayette Clinic aggression project. Unfortunately, many of the moral and legal dilemmas posed by this case in particular, and medical experimentation on institutionalized populations in general, remain unresolved. One point, for example, which the Detroit psychosurgery case did not clarify was what the state's role should be in supporting medical treatment programs designed to ameliorate aggressive, violent, or otherwise antisocial behavior by either invasive or noninvasive means. Undoubtedly, the court's decision in *Kaimowitz* v. *Department of Mental Health* will greatly influence the course of future debate over psychosurgery and behavior modification.

NOTES

1. Jo Thomas and Dolores Katz, "Surgery May Cure—or Kill—Rapist," *Detroit Free Press*, January 7, 1973, sec. A, pp. 1, 4, 5.

2. The Medical Committee for Human Rights is a national organization of medical professionals interested in improving health care delivery systems and community health programs. The petition and complaint was filed on the behalf of those members associated with the Ann Arbor and Detroit chapters.

3. *Kaimowitz* v. *Department of Mental Health,* Petition and Complaint, Civil No. 73-19434-AW (Cir. Ct., Wayne County, Mich., 1973), pp. 12-13.

4. *Kaimowitz* v. *Department of Mental Health,* Opinion, Civil No. 73-19434-AW (Cir. Ct., Wayne County, Mich., July 10, 1973), pp. 8-9.

5. For a more detailed legal analysis of this case, the reader is referred to John R. Mason, *"Kaimowitz* v. *Department of Mental Health*: A Right To Be Free From Experimental Psychosurgery," *Boston University Law Review* 54(March 1974): 301-339.

6. Vernon H. Mark and Frank R. Ervin, *Violence and the Brain* (New York: Harper & Row, 1970).

7. It has been hypothesized that the correlation between abnormal electrical activity in deep brain structures and certain behavioral dysfunctions may best be studied by implanting electrodes directly into the brain. Unfortunately, the diagnostic gains in terms of sensitivity and accuracy are counterbalanced by the serious medical risks associated with stereotactic surgery. Electroencephalography (EEG) is considered to be a standard and far less invasive means of recording electrical abnormalities in the brain, although the results may prove equivocal under certain circumstances. Court testimony and more recent reports reveal a heated debate among neurologists as to when depthelectrography is indicated as a diagnostic procedure. While some view the presence of chronic epilepsy, refractory to anticonvulsant medications, as the sole criterion, others wish to include patients suffering from severe behavioral disturbances as well. In any case, the correlation between abnormal electrical activity in the amygdaloid region of the limbic system and its role in precipitating uncontrollable aggression has not yet been established.

8. Ernst A. Rodin, "A Neurological Appraisal of Some Episodic Behavioral Disturbances with Special Emphasis on Aggressive Outbursts." Amicus Curiae Exhibit 3 dated March 27, 1973, p. 15. Presented at the Winter Conference of Brain Research in Colorado, January 1971.

9. According to testimony, the State Department of Mental Health was reluctant to release these few remaining patients in light of more recent evidence of serious and potentially dangerous behavioral dysfunctions.

10. Doe had been committed to Ionia in 1955 under the special CSP statute following an alleged rape and murder of a student nurse. On two occasions prior to the May 1972 meeting, he had been sent to Lafayette Clinic at Yudashkin's request for EEG studies which revealed the presence of borderline electrical abnormalities but no conclusive evidence of temporal lobe epilepsy.

11. Ernst A. Rodin, M.D., memo to Jacques S. Gottlieb, M.D., "Results of Discussions Held in Regard to Aggression Surgery," August 9, 1972. Amicus Curiae Exhibit 4 dated March 27, 1973, p. 8.

12. J. S. Gottlieb and Ernst A. Rodin, "Proposal for the Study of the Treatment of Uncontrollable Aggression at the Lafayette Clinic" (1972 revision). Plaintiff's Exhibit A, p. 3.

13. Ibid.

14. Elliot B. Luby, M.D., March 27, 1973, pp. 1-3. *Kaimowitz* v. *Department of Mental Health*, Testimony.

15. Gottlieb and Rodin, "Proposal for the Study," pp. 9-10.

ROBERT C. NEVILLE, Ph. D.

4 / Zalmoxis or The Morals of ESB and Psychosurgery

This Thracian told me that in these notions of theirs, which I was just now mentioning, the Greek physicians are quite right as far as they go, but Zalmoxis, he added, our king, who is also a god, says further, "that as you ought not attempt to cure the eyes without the head, or the head without the body, so neither ought you to attempt to cure the body without the soul. And this," he said, "is the reason why the cure of many diseases is unknown to the physicians of Hellas, because they disregard the whole, which ought to be studied also, for the part can never be well unless the whole is well." For all good and evil, whether in the body or in the whole man, originates, as he declared, in the soul, and overflows from thence, as if from the head into the eyes. —Plato, *Charmides* [p. 103].[2]

ANY spectacular invention bearing on man's health or behavior excites interest in its moral implications and in the values it affects. Electrical stimulation of the brain (ESB) and psychosurgery are no exceptions. But excited interest and accurate discernment of the real ethical issues are by no means the same thing. The first task of the ethical philosopher, therefore, is to locate the right problems so that the resources of the sciences and humanities can be properly focused.

In one sense, behavior control through physical manipulation of the brain (PMB) has most of the moral and value problems of any major medical procedure. When are risks justified? How is consent obtained? Who gives consent? What is *informed* consent? Is experimentation justified outside the context of a reasonable belief the procedure will be therapeutic? Is it legitimate to experiment on someone with the expectation the experiment will not succeed therapeutically, in hopes of developing sure techniques of helping people in the future? How is normalcy to be defined for therapy? What rights does a person have as a person, over and above being a medically interesting body or behavior? How does the technique determine the relationship between the patient and his doctors, nurses, medical staff, family, and so on? Who pays? How does this technology affect the distribution of money and resources for medical care? Who makes decisions on medical procedures? How are the costs and benefits in various qualities of life to be measured for the patient? For his family? For the society? Questions like these are not unique to techniques like ESB and psychosurgery; still, they are real questions for those fields.

Similarly, behavior control through PMB is involved in all the moral problems of *behavior control as such*. What kinds of behavior should be controlled? Pathological kinds? Undesired kinds? Whose behavior is controlled? Who controls? Who decides who controls? How does behavior control affect freedom and dignity? What are the costs of gaining self-control? What social interests justify social controls? What instruments of control are warranted to serve the interests of society?

Are there any ethical problems that arise *only* in the context of the modification of behavior through PMB? There would seem to be two sorts.

First, the brain is much closer than other body organs to what we take to be the center of behavior. Whereas we can conceive the body generally to be a kind of environment for the person, there is seemingly a peculiar intimacy between the brain and the person. Problems having to do with a person's rights over his own person are intensified when brain-modifying techniques are brought into play.

Second, because of the directness of control over thought and behavior, techniques manipulating the brain raise questions about the general image of man. The kind of being man is becomes an important question in this field in a way it would not be for techniques treating liver disease or even for behavior control methods employing, say, information media. A strategy for articulating the ethical issues of behavior control through direct manipulation of the brain must move through all these levels.

Environment and Brain

Is there anything that distinguishes behavior control through PMB from all other forms of behavior control? Most forms of behavior control work by manipulating the environment of the person to be controlled. Behaviorism's "operant conditioning" is an obvious example. But controls through media and information, through institutions and socialization processes, even through most forms of psychotherapy (especially those in which there is much talk) work this way, too. On the other hand, ESB, psychosurgery, and chemotherapy work through modifying the state of the brain directly. Electroshock therapy and some kinds of conditioning in which an environmental cue (e.g., a picture of a frosty dry martini) is related to a physiological control device (e.g., an emetic) are borderline cases between environment and nervous system. Is there any special significance to the difference between behavior control through the environment and that through the brain?

Some people, especially those greatly impressed with economic metaphors for metaphysics, would claim that a person owns or possesses his body in a unique way. Whereas his environment, perhaps even his hair and fingernails, legitimately might be alienated from him for good social reasons, his body, especially the irreplaceable brain and nervous system, are more nearly inviolable in a moral sense. "Inviolable" means the society cannot do anything to the person's body without his consent. Because the "consent" model here is economic, it supposes a working distinction between the owning consentor and the owned goods about which consent is given. Such a distinction is plausible in cases of consent to leg amputations, for instance. But it becomes problematic in cases of consent to psychotherapeutic procedures when the patient is not in a position to give or withhold consent. (This is abstracting for the moment from the problem of *defining when* a mental patient is in fact in a position to be able to give responsible consent.) In cases like these (and analogous ones, such as when the patient is unconscious) we look to the nearest adult kin for giving or withholding consent. The rationale here cannot be quite the economic one, since the kin do not own the patient. Asking for consent from kin has more to do with the supposition that they would have a fairly pure interest in deciding on the best welfare of the patient, sympathizing with him more than would be possible for harried medical people. Furthermore, although the kin usually lack the firsthand medical expertise, they might have a certain kind of privileged information, based on their knowledge of the patient's special beliefs, ambitions, and so on, which enables them to make guesses about what he would choose, were he able. In general, our practice regarding consent does not follow the economic metaphor consistently. We do not ask consent, for instance, of the patient's insurance company or of those who would become executors of his estate upon his death or incompetence. The rationale for consent practices is to be sought elsewhere.

Suppose we say, cognizant of the consent problem, that a person's body, even (especially) his brain, is itself a special environment for the person. Although this is perhaps an unfamiliar conception, it allows us to articulate a rationale for our practices regarding consent (although not justifying them in detail). It also allows us to formulate the distinction between environment and brain as one between an external kind of environment and an internal one, with appropriate differences.

The Brain as Environment for the Self

The brain can be viewed as an environing medium for the activities of the human self. It both conducts the world to activities of decision and enjoyment, and conducts decisions and human responses to public expression back in the world. The brain and nervous system provide perceptions of the world to be enjoyed and acted upon, perceptions that would not be possible without the complex and regular system of transmission. Far more important, the brain conducts culture, in all its manifold forms, to the self; the culture is learned in situations of overt behavior, but it is organized and stored for human use by the brain. No less important than these "afferent" functions of the brain as environment are its "efferent" functions. If a decision is made, the brain must organize the various nervous activities to carry it out, or at least to get the body moving. Similarly, the brain is the medium through which enjoyments and sufferings become gleams or grimaces upon the face. Whatever one's philosophical view of the freedom of decision and the spontaneity of enjoyment, it is desirable that the brain be quite regular and trustworthy in its environing functions. We want valid perceptions, accurate and efficiently organized memories, economical ways of acting upon decisions and expressing feelings. Although there is no rhetorical value in calling these brain functions "mechanical," we do want them to be regular and trustworthy, and also subject to being reset according to our wishes.

But what is the self that can be in such an environment? If we define the human person or self in terms of what we prize as especially valuable in human life (a safe enough procedure for a start, since we prize human selfhood above practically everything else and probably prize everything essential in that selfhood), the following seem to be essential: conscious feelings of and about the world and oneself; symbolic referring and inferring; an ability to judge the fitness of propositions by contextual appropriateness, conformity to rules, and evidence; an ability to determine actions by adopting a set of values to govern behavior; an ability to interpret the actions of one's body as coherent according to some ideals of one's personal identity through time; an assessment of things, including oneself, according to norms; an orientation of oneself in the world according to some reflection about the nature of that orientation—weeping, shuddering, laughing, praying, loving, and enjoying in little things and in ecstasy, each in the appropriate context. Many other characteristics could be listed as important to the self. Each one depends on the body, especially the brain and nervous system, both as a context in which to happen and a medium through which to be expressed.

But what is the "self" that performs all these human activities? If one begins with the conception of a self as a tiny organism inhabiting the nervous system, as platelets inhabit the circulatory system, that question cannot receive a sensible answer. We should rather conceive the self as a series of events taking place in the environment of the brain, and through that in the larger world environment. In one sense, of course, the event-series is a sequence of physical brain events, connected by various neurological regularities to other brain events in the environment. But the important thing about the brain events constituting the human self is not their physical relations but their emotional, logical, symbolic, interpretive, and intentional relations. These latter are the kinds of connections important for human selfhood. For physical brain events to be able to be related in these human ways, over and above the ordinary chemical relations of brain cells, requires the specific complex environment of the human brain. A good answer to the question, "What is the self that has the brain for its environment?" is, the sequence of events of human experience, related in ways that make human experience significant. The self is not something nonphysical, or something physical in the brain that is not part of the brain. It is rather various brain events the most interesting connections of which are not of neurons but of human meanings. From a purely physical standpoint, the self jumps around the brain, from frontal lobe to thalamus to occipital lobe. From the standpoint of the person the self is an advancing series of interpretive events, perceiving, willing, filling the brain with a culture of memories. Each event in the career of the self takes the other brain events, antecedent, contemporary, and subsequent, as its environment.

Consent

How does this make sense of our practices of locating responsibility for consent? The general principle would be something like this. A being sustained by and acting through an environment has a privileged right to profit from that environment. He values it directly in a self-referential way as the condition for his own existence. Therefore, a person directly values his own brain. Another person might value the first person's brain indirectly as a condition for that first person; he might also value the first person's brain as an instrument or work of art having a scientific interest. However, the outsider's existence would not depend on that environment in the direct way the person depends on his own brain. Because of the direct dependence of the person on his own brain, we say he should have first claim over what happens to it; in ordinary circumstances no one else would be in a position to claim that his own existence depends on another person's brain. This same principle of respecting the self-referential dependence of someone on his environment explains the high value many people put on democracy; it is preferable that a social group control the modifications of its own social structure.

If a person is not in a position to give or withhold consent about a proposed direct manipulation of his brain, we look for consent from people we expect to be most likely to prize a person's brain as the environment for *his* human experience. We tend to distrust doctors looking for experimental subjects, insurance agents looking for financial advantage, and so on. The nearest kin seems the most likely candidate, and surely is the easiest class to name in a legal rule. We shall return to the question of consent below.

Internal and External Environments

What is the difference, then, between the brain as environment for human experience and the more external environments? There are many differences, with practical moral consequences. Two will be mentioned here.

1.   First, the brain is a constant and regular environment. A person can leave one external environment for another quite different. Even some parts of his body can be exchanged for artificial or transplant parts or organs. But the association between a person's mental activity and his brain is constant and intimate. From this it follows, as a practical consequence, that modifications of the brain intimately affect personal identity more than

nearly anything else. This is at the heart of the special power of behavior control techniques that manipulate the brain.

Consider the following. We all recognize how important the external natural and social environment is for one's identity insofar as that is articulated through symbol systems and particular meanings; a modification of the environment can modify behavior through vast systematic symbolic changes. More intimately, a person's bodily environment can be modified through the amputation of a limb or severing of a nerve; this alters a person's kinesthetic identity, and the kinesthetic dimension underlies and conditions the person's basic orientation to at least the physical aspects of the external environment. A modification of the brain itself is even more intimate, and the effects of such a modification on the person's identity can be even more pervasive in the whole of identity than nearly any other kind of modification.

The moral of this is that ESB and psychosurgery (and also chemical means of behavior control) should be undertaken with the greatest awareness of potential pervasive effects of the procedure on the person's whole identity. We should not ask merely whether an amygdalectomy eliminates the capacity for certain forms of aggression. We should ask instead what are the total effects on a person's identity of having the capacity for those forms of aggression removed? This example even assumes that the procedure has no direct effects other than eliminating those forms of aggression.

The moral point here is intended to counteract the attitude that might be derived from Perry London's[3] defense of the "machine model of man." His main thesis is that man is a complex organism whose parts interact according to regular natural laws, like a machine. Although the rhetoric of machinery may be unnecessarily inflammatory, no quarrel is to be raised with respect to his claims about regularity in bodily functions. If there are spontaneous (nonregular) behavior events, those are precisely the ones behavior control cannot manipulate, in principle. The quarrel is rather with the practical attitudes likely to be generated by the image of man as machine, attitudes leading one to think we can alter one part of a man's brain without affecting a great deal else, like replacing a cog in a machine with a different part performing the same function. The view of man as a system of interconnected and systematically functioning parts is misleading. He should be viewed in terms of a series of nested environments, with each (relatively) external environment being humanly interesting in terms of the (relatively) internal environments, the brain being the most internal environment, filtering all messages in and out. London takes the humanistic or holistic view to be the alternative to his machine model. While not affirming the causal metaphysics he attributes to that alternative, the nested environment model suggests concepts of identity structure and causal alteration of identity somewhat more like the holistic view than the machine model. At any rate, it is very dangerous (others things being equal) to undertake modification of selective behavior symptoms by direct manipulation of the brain without taking into account ramifications on basic identity. This problem is far more serious for techniques physically manipulating the brain than for operant conditioning, control of information, and most other techniques of behavior control.

2. Second, the brain as an environment is too close to a person for him to be able to respond to modifications of it with his human, cultured resources. What this means is that he has no way of coping consciously with the procedures manipulating him. As a consequence, it is very difficult for there to be a process of gradual adjustment whereby the person can incorporate the modifications of his behavior with some personal integrity. One moment he is his old self, the next moment a new self, and he just has to lie there and take it.

This contrasts with most other forms of behavior control. In educational control, for instance, both the conveying of information and the structuring of the learning environment are such that a person copes with the modifications increment by increment, never going through massive behavior shifts. In higher education the ideals of behavior modification usually involve a kind of dialectic whereby a person chooses to do what will modify his behavior (e.g., read a book) for reasons he himself approves. The moral responsibility of the teacher is to provide good reasons the worth of which can be seen. Something not quite so free-spirited takes place in the transference operative in psychoanalysis, but still the modification of behavior involves doubling back on the personality and assimilating new elements, not shocking its whole structure. Operant conditioning, in principle, is supposed to deal with limited and circumscribed changes which themselves can be integrated into new patterns of behavior in limited increments. One could even argue that the influence of behavior-modifying drugs can be assimilated step by step because the effects of drugs wear off and treatment can be suspended if the alteration is too great. ESB and psychosurgery, the latter more than the former, produce changes that are massive and discontinuous. One's response to stimulation and the probe are not within the environment of personal control. Except for the few possibilities of control of the autonomic nervous system, a person's control is exercised in far more external environments.

The practical consequence of this fact is that, other things being equal, PMB should be undertaken only in psychotherapeutic contexts in which the patient can be helped to adjust his self-understanding and historical continuity to the new behavior forced upon him. In some contexts it might be valid to say "Let the buyer beware," but it makes no sense to say "Let the lobotomee beware!"

The concern for personal identity and the concern for a human appropriation of personality changes in a context of unique patient helplessness are moral considerations arising from the *special nature of the brain* as the locus of modifying activity. Another set of moral considerations arises in light of the problem of *the purposes served by behavior control techniques* directly manipulating the brain.

Purposes of Control—Therapeutic

At the present time most of the practice of electrical brain stimulation and psychosurgery is aimed to be therapeutic, in contexts in which the subject is taken to be a patient with a pathological disorder. It might be argued that some forms of therapy, for example, for broken legs or skin fungi, have no serious moral dimensions. But this cannot be said for therapeutic procedures regarding mental diseases. It especially cannot be said for procedures directly manipulating the brain, and for just the reasons of affecting identity and the capacity to appropriate humanly the changes in one's life detailed in the preceding section. How do the moral problems arise?

It would be an extravagance of indignation to complain about the use of brain manipulation procedures on the back ward cases for whom the only alternative is to spend the duration of their lives strait-jacketed in padded cells, ranting or dumb, with no evidence of human consciousness or feeling. Doubtless there are cases in which the risks involved in ESB and psychosurgery, even at their worst realizations, are far preferable to the alternatives. Of course it is possible to question *why* the only alternatives are the strait jacket versus the electrode, but this is a question of economics and politics.

Moving beyond the back ward cases, the moral perplexities get sticky. Suppose a patient were to walk into a hospital and request an ESB or psychosurgical procedure for ends of his own. Does the fact that the patient requests a procedure likely to produce the results he desires eliminate the issue of the moral propriety of performing the procedure? Given our usual *economic model* of freedom and morality, we would be inclined to say, "Give the customer what he wants." If it turns out that what he wants and gets is a real disaster, both penalty and fault lie with the customer. But suppose a person took seriously the biblical injunction that if a member of the body offends, cut it off; suppose a person requests amputation of his hands to cure kleptomania, or amputation of his penis to cure lascivious thoughts (remember Hemingway's story, "God Rest You Merry, Gentlemen"). Most doctors would be disinclined to accede to the requests. Their feeling would be that such procedures would result in unnecessary abnormality; what the customer wants is abnormal, unnatural, and unhealthy.

Defining the Normal

It seems impossible to discern the appropriateness of medical procedures without some conception of normality. Yet normality

97

is notoriously difficult to define. Normality can be defined with fair success within a closed system in terms of the harmony of interrelated functioning parts. In this sense, a blood clot blocking blood flow to a certain part of the brain is abnormal because it upsets the harmonious functioning of the brain in the body. But the important element of this approach is having a clear idea of the proper functioning of the closed system. There is nothing abnormal about blood clots blocking the flow of blood when they become wedged in constricted spaces—the laws of simple plumbing explain that. But we tend to think there is something unnatural in a man's paralysis resulting from a stroke. We have an idea of a whole, normal, natural, or healthy organism.

Behavior, however, which is the way an organism functions with respect to an external environment, is very difficult to describe in terms of the natural or normal. Unlike the circulatory system in the body, a man in society does not operate in a closed environment. Of course, we can construe mental health merely as adjustment to the social context, never questioning the social environment itself. This was the medically oriented reaction of some psychoanalysts to the problem of defining the ends of psychotherapy. But society is not closed. It is continually being reformed, and often according to ideals that call into question its basic structures. Psychological misadjustment (from the viewpoint in which society's habits are taken as legitimate norms) may in fact be adaptive behavior in light of the desired changes. One need not follow the line of *The Radical Therapist* to see that depression, frustration, anger, and even violence might be properly adaptive mechanisms.

The problem of defining the normal is especially acute in cases in which procedures of ESB or psychosurgery are considered. Probably the most widespread use of those procedures is to control aggression. But what is the role of aggression in human life? This depends on variations in the social situation. Man's genetic endowment gives him neurological control mechanisms to restrain or unleash aggression relative to age-old and relatively steady environmental factors. But modern society presents new, rapidly changing, and widely variable factors relevant to aggression that the genetic controls are too slow to meet. If the "territorial imperative" hypothesis is correct, an automobile driver would be acting naturally if he tried to run an alien vehicle off the road. Uniform driving laws, and the common habits they instill, can be viewed as attempts to make all vehicles smell like they belong to the local herd. The other side of the coin is that some of the genetic restraints on aggression might be misplaced. Our genetic endowment may approve a certain ritualized aggression in establishing a social pecking order, but it restrains behavior within the authority structure so established. This is certainly not a democratic heritage! If the democracy we approve by rational consideration is a worthy ideal, then women ought to be more openly aggressive against men, oppressed groups against their oppressors, and the ruled against the ruler. In a democratic society, restraints against aggression should respect social procedures and the prudence of political organization, not persons with power or its authoritarian symbols. Mental health regarding aggression cannot be defined without taking into account political and sociological factors. To the extent this consideration is true, medical doctors, with respect to their training, are lacking the expertise to define mental health; given the alleged hierarchical and paternalistic social understanding of doctors as a social class, doctors might be a positive hindrance to the definition of health.

Symptoms for behavior control other than aggression raise similar questions regarding normality. Take psychosurgery for homosexuality, for example. A young male Spartan in the days of Socrates who refused to take a male lover before he took a wife, on grounds of the unnaturalness of homosexuality, would have been thought definitely queer, and also unpatriotic. There are subgroups in our own society in which economics and friendship are such that homosexuality is the preferred adaptive mode.

The closed system organism is not satisfactory for defining the normal or natural. Perhaps those words should be given up as too much tied to the organism way of thinking. But we do need some handy images for defining what is "the good" for some person. Perhaps "health" connotes a personal norm that is relative to environmental differences.

From "Normal" to "Healthy"

In some sense, a person is healthy when he is physically and mentally equipped to make the best of his environment. The obvious truth in this statement is that the physical and mental conditions of health vary with significant changes in the environment; the genetically determined aggression controls appropriate for the savage hunter are unhealthy in modern urban society. But what does the rest of the statement mean? Suppose for the moment we hold the variables in the environment still, accepting the sociophysical environment as conventionally fixed, and look at variations in the individual.

1. A person is healthy if he can prosper in his environment. But what environment? Here we tend to have two divergent ideals. On the one hand we prize *flexibility*. A person should be able to prosper in several environments, or his overall environment should include many variations, from hot to cold, town to country, intimate to organizational, and so on. Therefore we prize physical and emotional make-ups that contribute to mobility. On the other hand, we prize investment in particularity, the ability to relate intensely to the environment, appropriating the cultural and physical resources richly and making return contributions that are directly relative to the environment, not merely generally creative. In a monolithic sociophysical environment flexibility would not be prized, since there is nowhere else to go. In a depersonalized social organization defined solely in terms of functional roles, investment in particularity would not be especially prized. But we prize both, and therefore healthy patterns of life in our society require maximizing both flexibility and particularity. It might seem that an advance toward one means a retreat from the other. But that is because we are unaccustomed to thinking explicitly of both as ideals and have not concentrated on finding patterns of life that can maximize both together.

What does this mean in practical terms for understanding the morality of ESB and psychosurgery? It is possible to judge the relative merits of the anticipated effects of some procedures in terms of their contributions to social mobility. It is also possible to judge in terms of their contributions to the intensity of particular involvements. But in fact those ideals ought to be

100

thought of together regarding their trade-offs, one to the other. A lobotomy might allow a person to function in society outside a mental hospital which otherwise would be his only possible environment. But the lobotomy might also cost the patient the ability to live intensely, to particularize the world he lives in. Measuring these costs is an empirical matter. But we must always revise our ideals, e.g., mobility, in terms of cost of their attainment to categorically related ideals, e.g., investments in particularity. Perhaps the healthiest thing for a patient is for the society to provide special environments (like mental hospitals) where a modicum of investment in particularity can be maintained.

2. Another aspect of the point that a person is healthy when he can make the best of his environment is *self-control*. The person is not only a factor in an environment, he is an agent in it. Without debating the issue of freedom, it is clear that we prize action that is self-controlled rather than controlled by others. Self-control is a very complex business, depending on a multitude of factors from genetic and cultural inheritance to environments tolerating and educating the exercise of self-control. But it seems that self-control is an ideal that itself is a pattern of compromise between two other ideals. On the one hand we want to set our own directions and ends; on the other we want to be able to appropriate the resources of the world to accomplish our ends. If a person chooses ends that are easy, relative to their accomplishment, self-control is not worth much. But if the ends are far out and appropriation of the resources requires great mastery of skill and knowledge, the self-control achieved by maximizing both is highly valuable.

Self-control is of great practical moment for techniques of behavior control that directly manipulate the brain. Aside from problems of controlling criminal behavior, we are tempted to think that the end of behavior control is self-control. A person can find help in ESB and psychosurgery if he cannot control his aggression, if he is subject to epileptic seizures, and so on. But some of those very same procedures exact a cost in other aspects of self-control through, for instance, loss of memory or sense of identity. Deliberation about the worth of some such procedure,

101

therefore, ought to be informed by a balanced and comprehensive view of the ideal of self-control.

3. A final dimension of the point that health consists in being able to make the best of one's environment has to do with *style*, and it is a matter of relating the first two points. In a rough sense, problems of relating to one's environment flexibly and with intensity have to do with enjoyment and fulfillment. Problems of self-control have to do with action. Action and enjoyment are inextricably bound together in our experience. Yet Western traditions have tended to conceive these in exclusive conceptual schemes. One focuses on action, and enjoyment is represented as something not very basic, or else enjoyment is basic and action merely instrumental. The German transcendental tradition of ethics has worried about the intrinsic morality of actions, with freedom and knowledge being defined in reference to law and obligation. The Anglo-Saxon tradition has concentrated on enjoyment and its costs, utilitarianism being the most famous theory of this sort. Each tradition is partial, and each calls forth the other. There is something true about both the categorical imperative and the principle of utility. But it seems that the price of making either one basic is the trivialization of the other.

The problem in concrete life reflected in the bifurcation of moral theories is how to reconcile concerns for good enjoyment with concerns for good action, or self-control. The reconciliation sought is not a theory, but a way of life discerning when it is important to attend to one kind of concerns, when to another. "Style" can be defined as a way of doing things with a characteristic pattern for evaluating things as important or trivial. A style pattern is not rigid; it often deals with novelties, and its parts evolve. It has more to do with habits of discerning importance than with remembered evaluations. Many factors enter the development of a style, such as expertise in a special field or methodology, familiarity with a special environment, or a sense of self and vocation. But however developed, a person needs a style to be healthy. He needs habits of distinguishing the important from the trivial. It is better to have a merely conventional style, one that is often objectively mistaken in its sense of importance, than to have no style at all.

A sense of style is such a general aspect of health it is difficult to see what bearing it has on the moral understanding of behavior control through ESB and psychosurgery. Yet if it is true, as was claimed earlier, that the deliberation about procedures in particular cases should consider the effects on the whole identity of the person, not just the effects on isolated symptoms, then the patient's style is very important. It characterizes some of the most general contours of his identity. But what difference does an ESB or psychosurgical procedure make to one's style? One of the reasons style is both hard to define and hard to control is that its variables are not so much in the external environments of overt actions, symbol systems, and the like, as in the inner environment of the brain. In other language, one might say that the stylistic factors in behavior are preconscious; we think the thoughts we do because of our styles more than we have the styles we do because of our thoughts. Style has to do with a sense of timing, a sense of prereflective connections, aversions and adversions. If you want to change someone's style, it would be very inefficient to do so by changing the things to which he has to respond, although this method is most respectful of the person's choice of style. The more efficient way is to change his brain. Although we have not the foggiest idea about how to change the brain to bring about a deliberate change in style, the regularities of style are in the brain. Therefore our very ignorance of how to control styles by changing the brain means that our manipulation of the brain, for whatever other reasons, is likely to alter a person's style. Effects upon style are among the most important effects to be examined in deliberating about whether to perform some procedure.

The discussion of this section has been aimed to elucidate the moral dimensions of the therapeutic purposes of behavior control that might be accomplished through ESB and psychosurgery. Philosophy, of course, cannot say what those procedures are competent to do. The point has been rather to think through the notion of therapy in the context of brain manipulation techniques. The discussion began with the idea that therapy should give the patient what he wants ("help me stop having aggressive rages"). It was seen that the limit to this economic model was that what the patient wants must be something normatively good, something normal or natural. But the difficulties in defining naturalness or normality outside the context of a closed system led us to attempt to define health as a norm. For the psychosocial purposes relative to behavior control through ESB and psychosurgery, we defined health in terms of the ability of a person to make the best of his environment. Flexibility versus investment in particularity, self-control, and general style were seen to be related dimensions of health defined this way.

An explicit limitation of our discussion should be recalled to mind, however. We assumed the factors of the environment were fixed and asked only about the problems of the individual in making the best of it. This was because we are considering only techniques for altering individual behavior. But we could have held the notion of the individual still, using "typical" people as examples, and asked how the environment could be altered so that the best to be made of it can be maximized. This is a political problem, not a medical one as that is usually conceived. There is, as everyone knows, a strong debate regarding where to spend our resources: shall they be used to advance individualized medical technology or to alter the social and physical environment? An even more important question, however, is whether the consideration of even the *medical* issues of health can be legitimate without the social and political dimensions of those issues being made explicit.

Purposes of Control—Social

At the present time, techniques of ESB and psychosurgery are employed mainly in therapeutic contexts. They are construed as techniques of behavior control when control is sought as a cure for illness. Behavior control is not an issue that is of interest only to doctors and patients, however. Society itself engages in many forms of behavior control, for many reasons. It needs control in education to keep the society's resources on tap; control of traffic to keep people, goods, and services moving; control over criminal behavior to protect the lives, property, and interests of its citizens.

It is conceivable that the techniques of ESB and psychosurgery can be employed for control in these and similar social areas. They are already being employed in other countries to treat cases of chronic criminal aggression and obsessive sexual behavior, and they are being taken seriously as full-scale alternatives to imprisonment and other traditional forms of punishment.

The morally important factor about socially imposed forms of control is that they are imposed. That is, the people controlled are coerced into submission to the forms of control. If they can be brought to desire the control, and therefore seek it just as if they were looking for therapy from a doctor so much the better. But want it or not, the control is forced upon them.

Let us suppose that certain behavior is socially necessary, and that we need to find the best form of control to guarantee that kind of behavior. Of course there are political considerations involved in choosing the kind of behavior deemed necessary, in establishing reasonable distinctions between desired and necessary behavior, and in distinguishing between modes of behavior required of all people, of a sufficient number of people, and of certain particular people. But suppose that some way or another, society makes these decisions. What considerations are important in its moral deliberation about whether to employ ESB and psychosurgery as means of control?

Society's interest is not prima facie to make the controlled individuals healthy: its interest is to bring about the desired behavior for the sake of the society. We would like to think that contributing to the health of our citizens is a means to socially necessary behavior, and no doubt it often is. But there is no necessary connection here. Sometimes things must be done to a person for the benefit of society that no one would think to be for the good of the person himself. Prisons are bad for people; yet some people must be put there to protect society from them. Amygdalectomies are dangerous, but they may be means to protect society from certain people, and they may be preferable to prisons (although this has yet to be shown).

Assuming that there is a social need to control certain behavior, the choice of means should be made by comparison of alternatives. If the alternatives regarding a criminal, for instance, are

105

prison versus a certain psychosurgical procedure, and there is no therapeutic justification for either, only that of protecting society, how does one choose between them? There seem to be three kinds of criteria: degree of guaranteed protection or efficiency, social cost, and personal respect.

Guaranteed Efficiency

If society is ever justified in exercising coercive control, it should make sure its necessary needs are fulfilled. This means, for instance, that if a man, convicted of a murder committed while in a rage of aggression, is a candidate for a psychosurgical procedure, the effectiveness of the procedure in preventing future rages must be assessed. The assessment is an empirical problem, of course, and it is very complicated since aggression is such a multifarious behavior trait. Presumably, however, even when we know much more than we do now, the best predictions will always carry with them a certain margin of error. But then by itself the margin of error in the prediction is meaningless for deliberation. It must be compared with the degree of protection afforded by imprisonment. After all, sentences of imprisonment are of finite length and the criminal can be returned to society. Even murderers can be given time off for good behavior. What is the likelihood that imprisonment will protect society from the aggressive rage in comparison with a psychosurgical operation? That is a complex empirical matter. The probable degree of success in achieving the socially necessary behavior is an important criterion in choosing the proper means.

Social Cost

Efficiency in attaining the socially necessary behavior must be weighed against social cost. That is, what price does society pay to sustain various forms of control? The social price of prisons, for instance, is very high indeed. They seem to make the bad men worse, corrupt guards and officials, deceive society into not looking at egregious social ills, and train criminals to do more efficient criminal work when they get out. Are there comparable social costs for ESB and psychosurgery? This is a matter that has received little attention so far, since we are only beginning to take these forms of control seriously. But there are undoubtedly some social costs in tax money, the development of a large class of practitioners, and so forth. Of course, the alternative with the least social cost may not have the acceptable level of efficiency. These two criteria must be balanced.

Personal Respect

In a democratic society, a third kind of criterion must be introduced, personal respect. That is, even in the case of control of a criminal, the criminal's humanity ought to be respected as much as possible. This criterion is reflected in our laws against cruel, unusual, and excessive punishments. In our present context, the criterion has to do with determining which of the alternatives does the most good or least harm to the person of the criminal. Within the limits of the criteria of efficient protection of society and of minimal social cost, control of criminal behavior should improve the criminal as much as possible. Bringing the criminal closer to health, in the senses discussed above, is the obvious improvement.

Society's interest in controlling behavior, in summary, is related to alternative methods of control (of which ESB and psychosurgery are potential candidates) in a complex way. Not only must one judge each candidate procedure in light of its alternatives, one must also balance out at least three kinds of criteria for judging the alternatives. This suggests that, although a candidate procedure may not score highest according to any single criteria, it might have the highest score in maximizing the three concerns together. This kind of moral deliberation is very difficult, but appropriate and necessary to the situation.

Who Controls?

There is an important and often neglected distinction between questions of who should make decisions about the use of behavior control procedures and questions concerning the criteria on which such decisions should be based. Most of our discussion has focused on criteria for making the decisions, abstracting from the problems of who has the right or obligation to decide (or refrain from deciding). Whoever makes the decision should want to make a wise one and should call in whatever experts might be helpful in advising him. In hospital procedures like those involved in ESB and psychosurgery, a prima facie duty of the hospital should be to lay out the dimensions of the problem and provide the expertise for whoever makes the decision.

The question of who makes the decisions, however, has equal importance from the moral point of view with the question of what criteria are to be employed in the decision. The spectacular aspects of new techniques of behavior control, in fact, come from the specter of the wrong forces gaining control.

Who Controls Therapeutic Purposes?

It does not seem to be controversial to begin with the acknowledgment that in cases of control for therapeutic purposes the patient himself should make the decision by giving consent. In cases where the patient is incapable of giving or withholding consent, it should be given by his personal proxy. There is nothing in the relation of the patient to the doctor or hospital staff that would put the decision in the hands of the doctor, without the patient's explicit authorization. Of course it might be argued that the very act of coming to the hospital—if this was done voluntarily and in consciousness of the consequences—constitutes authorization of the hospital staff or doctor to make the decision. It is doubtful, however, in cases involving potential ESB and psychosurgery, that the consequences of hospital admission can ever be predicted with sufficient clarity for this argument to hold. Therefore consent rests with the patient or his proxy.

The consent must be genuinely *informed,* however. If it is not, a distinction develops between who consents to or decides to use a procedure, on the one hand, and who controls on the other. If the consent is not informed, the procedure is approved by the consenter but the results are either controlled by those performing the procedure or not controlled by anybody.

Consent can fail to be informed when either of two conditions holds.

1.   It might be the case that the procedure in question has unpredictable consequences. No procedure can be analysed predictively with 100 percent accuracy; but the results of some procedures can be predicted well enough, and the range of possible error stated clearly enough, so that the decision to use the procedure (or not to use it) can be reasonably informed. Procedures that are "experimental" are those for which it is problematic that informed consent can be given. It is dubious that informed consent is possible when the doctor can say only that possible results fall within a wide range of alternatives. In these cases no one would be in a position to give or withhold consent, and the procedure should not be employed. The only exception to this—one that restores the possibility of informed consent—is when it is clear that none of the possible outcomes of the procedure would be as bad as refraining from the procedure or employing an alternative procedure. In this case the decision is between the outer limits of possible outcomes of the procedure and its alternatives. But if the outer limits cannot be established, or the alternatives conceived, then the consent cannot be informed, and the procedure cannot be undertaken with confidence in its moral propriety.

2.   It might be the case that through negligence, disrespect for the lay mind, or inability to communicate, the doctors fail to provide the consenter with information they themselves possess. The problems involved here are very significant from a sociological point of view, and they extend far beyond considerations of consent for procedures of ESB and psychosurgery. Short of a general reformation of the medical profession and its educational system, the suggestion of a hospital board of review below is a stop-gap check on this kind of failure to obtain informed consent.

Consent should not only be informed but also *rational.* This means that the decision maker must not only be apprised of the consequences of the alternatives, he must also be able to approach the decision in a normal frame of mind, enabling him to act with maximum sensitivity to the real values involved. We would be disinclined, for instance, to allow a mother suffering from severe postpartum depression to make decisions concerning procedures to sustain the life of a deformed child. In cases of mental patients who are candidates for ESB and psychosurgery it is especially difficult to decide whether they are rational enough to decide these things. The famous case of Thomas the engineer, patient of Drs. Ervin, Mark, and Sweet, illustrates the point: when under the influence of calming electrical stimulation he consented to psychosurgical procedures aimed at destroying certain brain cells, but when the effects of the stimulation wore off he refused consent. When was he in his "right mind"? Fortunately, the staff persuaded him to give consent when he was not under the influence of recent stimulation. But then, perhaps he was under undue persuasive pressure. Given the oft-noted tendency of patients to become psychologically dependent on their doctors, it is very difficult to determine when consent is right-minded or rational.

If it is so difficult to determine when consent is informed and rational, then there should be some agency to decide whether consent in various cases is duly formed. It would seem to be advisable for each hospital where procedures of ESB and psycho-surgery are performed to have boards of consent review (a) whose members are not members of the team treating the specific case and (b) whose members include legal and moral experts. These review boards would pass in each instance on whether consent had been properly given (or withheld) and whether the consenter had been given adequate information and was in a proper frame of mind to make a reasonable decision. This suggestion would greatly complicate the life of a hospital; but it is more than worthwhile to protect the integrity of the patient, and to protect both the hospital staff and proxy consenters from actions that on reflection cannot be approved. Since emergencies are not common in the control techniques being considered here, such a review board would seem to be a plausible check on who controls.

Two objections to this analysis should be noted and dealt with.

First, what happens in a case where neither the patient nor his relatives is in a position to give informed consent, by virtue of hysteria or invincible ignorance, and yet the procedure is well understood, perhaps even standard, and such that any reasonable man would consent to it (or withhold consent)? Presumably the hospital consent review board would disqualify any of the principals, including relatives, from giving or withholding consent. Would we be committed, on the analysis given above, to denying permission to perform the reasonable procedure? Would this not be denying a patient means to recovery and health on the absurd reason that he and his relatives were not in a position to give consent? No. The doctors would still have the right to appeal to a legal court to overrule the judgment of the review consent board; or rather, the court would appoint a reasonable proxy to give consent, one acceptable to the consent review board. Just as doctors can now go to court to overrule a particular consent decision, they could also ask the court to appoint a proxy consenter acceptable to the consent review board.

The second objection is that this concentration on the niceties of consent undermines a legitimate interest in experimentation. Psychosurgery, ESB, and a variety of related techniques of behavior control offer great promise of being able to contribute to a more civilized society, as Delgado has pointed out in his book, *Physical Control of the Mind*.[1] But these techniques must be improved by experimentation before they can even begin to realize their promise. No one would argue that experimentation should be done without proper respect for the patient being experimented on. But the future generations who might profit from the experimentation have a logical and moral claim to influence the decisions in particular cases. Specifically, they have a right to insist that the criterion of "most likely to increase knowledge" be included among the various therapeutic criteria in deciding what procedure to employ. The patient himself, or his consenting proxies, cannot be expected to feel the weight of this claim by future generations, and therefore the consent requirement ought not to be allowed a veto power over decisions regarding treatment, according to this objection.

Against this objection several things need to be said. First of all, it is not clear that future generations have a claim on what we do that is anything like a moral balance to the claims of living people. Second, if there is indeed a distinction between the knowledge-productiveness of alternative procedures, why doubt that the patient himself would not take this into consideration in his

111

consent deliberation? Of course, if there were a wide difference between safe and unsafe procedures, he would be expected to incline toward the former; but so would anyone else, in the interest of prudential therapy. Third, the patient is a person, not an experimental animal, and nearly everyone agrees that persons ought to be treated as ends in themselves, not as means only. An experimental procedure, although its interest in advancing knowledge treats the patient as a means, may very well treat the patient as an end in himself if the procedure is also the best for his health. But if the procedure is not best for his health—and this is the only case in which it becomes interesting to set the interest in advancing knowledge up against the interest of therapy—then it detracts from treating the patient as an end in himself. To the extent special pleading is allowed for the experimental interest, the patient is dehumanized. It is difficult to see how future generations can have a claim on a person entailing his dehumanization.

Since it is the case that doctors and related scientists have a special interest in furthering the experimental research aspects of their work, it is very important for consent review boards to be watchdogs for a biased influence over the consent process. Doctors quite unconsciously can present the experimental procedures in an unduly favorable light because of their hope that consent will be given in that direction. Perhaps it is impossible to be absolutely neutral in the presentation of possibilities directly related to one's research interests. This is why the consent review board should be composed of people *not* part of the hospital group that would do the therapy.

This brings the discussion to a final point concerning the most important question in therapeutic procedures: Who controls? In philosophical language, the discussion of consent above has made reference to a principle of *privacy* and to a principle of *public life*.

It has been maintained, in effect, that procedures directly touching the brain for therapeutic purposes of modifying behavior should be subject to the private decision of the patient. If the person cannot give consent himself, we turn for consent to those most likely to empathize with his private concerns and point of view. This principle of privacy can be roughly formulated as follows: What is done to a person's brain for therapeutic or other purposes is his private matter, over which he alone should exercise control.

On the other hand, our society has come to regard this right of private control over one's brain as such an important matter that it supports a *public guarantee* of this right. At least our legal and medical practice has been moving in this direction, and the suggestion of instituting consent review boards in all hospitals performing neurosurgical procedures of this sort is at least one form this public guarantee might take. If they include ethicists and lawyers as well as doctors, they would be somewhat immune from the biases of doctors; yet they would be close enough to the actual procedures to be of particular help.

From an historical and sociological point of view, the question of how a society comes to regard some value as a *private right* to be guaranteed by a *public agency* is an interesting one. Likely it has to do with an evolving social consciousness of priorities and degrees of value. Hardly anything has proved itself to be as valuable as the forms by which a human being is a person, and choosing what happens to oneself as a person is one of the most important forms of personhood. Because of the intimate character of the brain as an environment for the person, we also value the privacy of choice about what effects the brain as an important form of personhood.

Private rights, however, have always been seen as limited by public social necessities. As discussed above, behavior often needs to be controlled for compelling social reasons, and sometimes in ways that are directly countertherapeutic. When techniques of behavior control are exercised out of social interests, we are again faced with the question: Who controls?

Who Controls for Social Purposes?

Fears of a "Brave New World" do not arise in a context of merely therapeutic deliberations about techniques of behavior control in individual cases. They arise rather in two contexts. On the one hand, it is to be feared that those *social interests* that would be expressed would be dehumanizing and enslaving. On the other hand, it is to be feared that forms of therapy *delivered in*

113

mass ways will be equally dehumanizing and enslaving. Because ESB and psychosurgery seem not to be mass-delivery systems of behavior control, at least not in the near future, the former is the greater context for concern here.

Suppose that ESB and psychosurgery in fact offer reasonable and preferable alternatives to imprisonment in the handling of criminals. The question here is who decides what behavior is criminal in such a form that it should best be dealt with by ESB or psychosurgery? Consider the "law-and-order" approach to this question. According to a large school of social commentators, the "law-and-order" philosophy really means "protect the social and economic status quo by blaming all criminal behavior on morally indigent individuals." The alternative, of course, is to levy heavy blame on certain social conditions that ought to be changed as a first priority. It can be argued that moral heroism is required to avoid criminal behavior if one is raised under certain unfavorable conditions, and we cannot expect moral heroism. However one feels about these political issues, it is clear that the "law-and-order" philosophy is a political position, not another name for the "true" and the "just." Whereas we have not discovered that ESB or psychosurgical procedures render a man law-abiding, they can render him docile. Yet if the ends defining criminal behavior ought to be opposed on moral and political grounds, the distribution and control of the power to render a man involuntarily docile is a grave problem. Of course the old power to incarcerate is not to be granted lightly, and our judicial system has a long and hard-won series of checks on that power. It might even be argued that when criminal behavior is unjustly defined and punished, it is better to have prisons than electrodes. After all, men retain their individual integrity at least for a while in prison. They might break out, and it can be argued that for the black community, for instance, the prison experience is sometimes a boon to developing political consciousness. At any rate, the empirical questions about the consequences of different forms of control must be investigated in detail.

Who controls the social forces of behavior control? This question allows no simple empirical answer. The moral question of who *should* control, however, has a simple beginning: the people

114

of the society. Defining the people, of course, is a difficult matter. But an initial practical conclusion is that society ought to address the question of how to render ESB and psychosurgical techniques of behavior control for social purposes subject to democratic control and review. This is a very general consideration, however, stemming from the fact that the definition of criminal behavior itself ought always to be under democratic review. Is there anything special about the control of the social use of ESB and psychosurgery?

It would seem that in many criminal cases where ESB or psychosurgery might be alternatives to incarceration, it would be possible to allow the convicted man to choose between them himself. In these cases, the moral problems would revert to those of consent.

It would also seem advisable to allow the convicted person, his family, or his lawyers, a right to appeal a sentence to submission of physical manipulation of his brain. There may be good reason to urge right of appeal of judicial sentencing in all cases. But there is something special about ESB and psychosurgery as "remedies" for crime: they not only protect the society (if they work), they alter the identity of the convict. If ESB or psychosurgery cannot be justified on therapeutic grounds as well as on grounds of protecting society, these procedures would violate the person's moral right not to be treated as a means only.

In brief, the potential new powers of behavior control for social purposes should alert us to one more desperate need to perfect the procedures and practices of democracy. In light of the long-recognized necessity that democracy take place in a context where important facts are disclosed in public, it should go without saying that the practices of ESB and psychosurgery should be made known, monitored faithfully, and regulated according to procedures of democratic check. This by no means entails that *government* is the sole agency of democracy; as Dewey pointed out, government is too often just another private party with special interests. Rather, the public and democratic monitoring and regulation of ESB and psychosurgery are more likely to flourish in a complex arrangement of differently organized groups: doctors, patients, lawyers, special interest groups, or even private watchdog organizations.

115

Conclusion

This chapter began with a quotation from Plato regarding the way in which health is a matter of the whole person, body and soul. That way in particular, according to Plato, consisted in the soul's being the unifying principle of the body, both in perceiving through it and acting through it. The surface theme throughout this chapter has been the various moral issues that arise due to the fact that the brain, the most intimate environment for the person himself, is subject to direct manipulation through ESB and psychosurgery. The deeper theme has been that our new ability to control behavior by manipulating this intimate environment calls for a new image of man himself. Some modest contributions to this new image have been suggested in the notion of the brain as environment and in the reinterpretation of health. At each stage in the discussion practical suggestions have been made regarding special problems and principles to judge by. But the final aim of this chapter greatly extends Plato's point (although he would have agreed with the extension): the unifying activity of the soul has little character of its own but is determined by its wider environments. The most concrete context for viewing the cure of the soul is politics. The moral issues raised by ESB and psychosurgery cannot be contained within medical ethics as they are usually conceived, but are in fact political problems. This is obvious in problems of controlling the controllers. It is perhaps less obvious but no less true when it comes to defining mental health. And it even is the case that the conservation of personal identity and integrity, the concern touched on at the beginning in the context of the consent issue, is the heart of political responsibility.

REFERENCES

1. Delgado, Jose M. R. *The Physical Control of the Mind.* New York: Harper & Row, 1969.
2. Hamilton, E. and Huntington, C., eds. *Plato: Collected Dialogues.* Bollingen Series 71. Princeton: Princeton University Press, 1961.
3. London, P. *Behavior Control.* Chap. 7. New York: Harper & Row, 1969.

HAROLD EDGAR, LL.D.

5 / Regulating Psychosurgery: Issues of Public Policy and Law

WORRYING about technological advance has become common. Yet the development of sophisticated techniques to control human behavior provokes this response to an exceptional extent. That is true even though promoters have proferred the techniques as potential solutions to problems such as violence that frighten everyone in our crime-conscious society. The number of violent crimes is increasing: more ominously, the damage that can be done by a few violent persons is augmented greatly by their access to the same sophisticated technology that serves us all. Society's most visible protection against such behavior, the criminal justice system, is widely perceived to be ineffective. Moreover, it relies upon solemnly condemning offenders, a stance that makes many people queasy because offenders are so often products of emotional and physical deprivations over which they had no control. Underestimating the attractiveness of therapeutic solutions to deviate behavior is folly.

Working against this desire to see crime go away is repulsion at mind control.[1] The possible political use of technology to control dissenting politics labeled deviant behavior is frightening. But the fears go deeper. Other medical developments, genetic surgery for example, may remake "Humanity" in ways far more significant

117

than anything aspired to by scientific behavior controllers. Few people believe themselves candidates for refabrication. By contast, behavior control threatens *us*. As mental illness is redefined to the point that much of the population may properly be called ill, the likelihood of being a recipient of the technology at the behest of well-meaning friends and loved ones increases. Indeed, a certain self-depreciation is required to believe that no one has any interest in controlling one's mind and behavior. "He's not worth controlling" is hardly a compliment, however true it may be. Moreover, that our thoughts and behavior may be controlled mechanically undermines a sense of ourselves as self-determined entities. If successfully developed, behavior control techniques will deflate self-conceptions, much as did Darwin and Copernicus in earlier times.

Because of this ambivalence about behavior control, psychosurgery became an issue. Four years ago, use of the term psychosurgery elicited quizzical stares. Now it has been the subject of state[2] and federal legislation,[3] Congressional hearings,[4] and a major public interest lawsuit.[5] This paper is an assessment of whether psychosurgery warrants special regulatory attention. My tentative answer is that it does, and perhaps uncautiously, I have stated some possible guidelines. I have done so as much to illustrate the number of distinguishable factors on which rules might turn as with any illusions that such rules are fully adequate. I should also make clear that, although a study of psychosurgery highlights regulatory inadequacies, most of the problem results from the fact that experimental surgery is still a laissez-faire business. After a brief discussion of some terminological problems, I shall elaborate on these themes.

Terminology

"Psychosurgery" means any operation designed to irreversibly lesion or destroy brain tissue for the primary purpose of altering the thoughts, emotions, or behavior of a human being. "Psychosurgery" does not include procedures which may irreversibly lesion or destroy brain tissues when undertaken to cure well-defined disease states such as brain tumor, epileptic foci, and certain chronic pain syndromes.[6]

118

Psychosurgery [is] the destruction of normal brain tissue for the control of emotions or behavior; or the destruction of abnormal brain tissue for the control of emotions or behavior, where the abnormal tissue has not been shown to be the cause of the emotion or behavior in question.[7]

Psychosurgery is defined as those operations currently referred to as lobotomy, psychiatric surgery, and behavioral surgery and all other forms of brain surgery if the surgery is performed for the purpose of the following:

1) Modification or control of thoughts, feelings, actions or behavior rather than treatment of a known and diagnosied physical disease of the brain;

2) Modification of normal brain function or normal brain tissue in order to control thoughts, feelings, action or behavior; or

3) Treatment of abnormal brain function or abnormal brain tissue to modify thoughts, feelings, actions or behavior when the abnormality is not an established cause for those thoughts, feelings, action or behavior.[8]

Psychosurgery is difficult to define usefully, and no common understanding of the term has developed. Everyone agrees that psychosurgery is brain surgery and destroys brain tissue. The destruction may be accomplished with primitive tools such as a modified ice pick, or with exceedingly complex ones, such as the nitrogen-cooled cannula. All such operations are irreversible in the sense that brain tissue, unlike skin, does not regenerate. Although that fact is insignificant in itself, it may lend support to the view that brain functioning is, for better or worse, substantially affected by major procedures.

All brain operations, however, inevitably destroy irreplaceable brain tissue. And while all psychosurgery involves brain procedures, the reverse is not true. No one deems removal of a brain tumor a psychosurgical procedure. Consequently, the hard problem is what makes some brain surgery "psycho" and the rest of it not. The three definitions I have set out, and indeed all those I have seen, focus on the motive with which the procedures are done: to alter thoughts, emotions, or behavior, behavior, or emotions or behavior, respectively. This mode of definition creates some difficulties for it prevents precise ascertainment of whether psychosurgery has taken place. One cannot tell simply by looking at what has transpired in the operating room. By itself, this objection to the definition is not compelling. Acts are constantly categorized by the motives which animate them; indeed, as Robert Michels noted, the only way to differentiate psychotherapy from

119

conversation is by reference to the parties' intent that therapy take place.[9] But definition in terms of motive is troublesome if, as in psychosurgery, motives are often mixed. For example, consider the case of an aggressive person who also shows evidence of epilepsy. Is an operation on such a person "psychosurgical" if the patient's aggression entered into the decision to operate, regardless of whether most neurosurgeons would regard the epileptic condition alone as warranting surgery?

A second definitional problem is the ambiguity of words like "behavior." In one sense everything an organism does is its behavior. Used so broadly, however, nearly all medical interventions are "behavior control" procedures, in that they are done to interfere with an organism's present or projected behavior. Brain tumors are removed because otherwise the patient will "fall down and die," or suffer other major interference with capacity to function. It would be malpractice to operate were the tumor not likely to have any effect on the patient's behavior in this broad sense. We do not swallow pills simply because we have viruses; medication is recommended only when a particular virus is affecting or is likely to affect the way we feel and can behave.

Perhaps most people would not regard "falling down and dying" as a statement about a person's behavior. Clearly, however, a brain operation destroying normal brain tissue in an effort to alleviate the shaking hands of a patient with Parkinson's disease is done to control "behavior" in a common sense of the word. As I understand it, this procedure is not deemed psychosurgery by neurosurgeons, and yet, unless behavior is taken narrowly, it seems covered by our three definitions. The second definition might exclude it because Parkinson's disease is a "well-recognized disease state," but that leaves the scope of psychosurgery to be resolved by one's understanding of what is "well-recognized." Is schizophrenia well-recognized?

Probably the definitions of psychosurgery intend "behavior" to connote less. The image is beating up a policeman, not shaking due to organic disease. But is the principle whether the behavior is "voluntary," and if so, what does that phrase mean? Is the distinction between behavior which is thought to be the product of conscious choice, and that which is either "compelled" or reflexive? Or, alternatively, is the distinction between "behaviors" whose "physical" cause is known, and those whose origins are shrouded in mystery, but must surely have some biochemical base? For example, consider a patient who reports himself to be experiencing intense pain. Is a brain operation to ameliorate that experienced pain a psychosurgical procedure if the patient has cancer, or is suffering pain in an amputated (phantom) limb, or if he simply says "Doctor, I hurt?"[10]

Failure to develop uniform usage of the term "psychosurgery" is no great hindrance to regulation, for if regulation is decided upon, the definitional issue may be by-passed by describing the regulated procedures in detail. But the fact that people commonly use the term "psychosurgery" in significantly different ways underlines an important point. It may be that these procedures are not sufficiently different from regular brain surgery to warrant special inquiry on grounds that they deal with the "psyche." The proper question may be simply whether or not such procedures are good surgery.

Thus I wish to put my principal emphasis on the regulation of innovative surgery within the context of regulation of experimental medicine generally. It is not the glamour issue presented by psychosurgery. We are not met here with the intersection of medicine and the penal system—the warden dressed up in doctor's whites. Even so, I believe the most crucial questions about public policy and psychosurgical techniques center upon the adequacy of our current modes of ascertaining whether medical procedures are effective in accomplishing the ends for which they are employed at appropriate levels of risk under the circumstances. The problem does not involve a frontal clash between social control and individual rights, but is a more complex one of protecting patients from unwarranted risks without either unduly hindering innovation or transforming the doctor-patient relationship from therapy to hypothesis-testing. These issues are present whether psychosurgery is performed on fully competent adults or violent offenders. But such issues have special importance, I believe, in programs in which social control is an element. If one examines the history of other efforts to substitute therapy for more traditional means of influencing social behavior, such as sexual psychopath laws or narcotics commitment laws, an overriding objection to them, aside from all questions of society's right to impose coercive therapy, is that the purported therapy does not work. Although I do not doubt the difficulty of the philosophical issues presented if these procedures do all their most vigorous proponents claim, the central problem for now is whether the regulatory mechanisms currently employed to answer such questions as whether and how they work, and to limit the damage to successive groups of patients if they do not work are adequate.

Regulation of Innovative Surgery

Innovative surgery is subject to little formal regulation. Although surgical innovations vary widely in terms of the risks they pose to patients, it is difficult to find any other area of social life in which people are permitted to subject others intentionally to comparable risks with so few formal mechanisms for oversight.[11] Innovative surgery can be very dangerous indeed, as is indicated both by the figures collected by Swazey and Fox on mitral valve surgery[12] and the more recent experience with heart transplant procedures.[13] Do not be misled: evaluating danger without regard to the patient's alternatives cannot answer whether procedures are justified. Nonetheless, it is startling to realize that, as a practical matter, the decision of whether to expose patients to a 70 percent chance of death on the operating table is confided to the discretion of the individual surgeon restricted only by informal and uncoordinated controls.

First, the major control mechanism, the threat of malpractice litigation, threatens inconvenience rather than substantial hazards for the surgeon who obtains "informed consent" by telling the patient all he knows. That is particularly the case when, as in psychosurgery, many of the perceived adverse consequences may be inevitable concomitants of the procedure rather than the rare bad result.

Second, peer group review of the work of individual surgeons at their institutions is limited. As I understand it, the usual concern of tissue review committees is whether a particular operation has been done properly and whether the diagnosis that prompted it was correct. The broader question of whether a particular type of operation ought to be done at all because other therapies promise better results is not typically within its jurisdiction. That question is answered, if at all, only on an ad hoc basis. Unless the innovation is undertaken as part of a funded research project, subject to Department of Health, Education and Welfare (HEW) rules requiring institutional review committees, there is no automatic necessity for a group of qualified experts to pass on the balance of risks and benefits accompanying it.

Third, no public agency is charged with the duty to review and approve surgical innovation. Innovations in drug therapies are under reasonably close control through the Food and Drug Administration (FDA). Innovations in surgical practice are not. Whether the differences between the two forms of therapy justify the gap in regulatory practice is doubtful.

Finally, and most importantly, procedures do not exist to ensure that the data necessary for anyone to judge properly the risks and benefits accompanying a particular procedure are collected and made available promptly.

Data Collection

I believe coordination of research efforts and data collection is a precondition to effective regulation of psychosurgery and desirable independent of any other regulation, and I shall therefore start my brief review of each of the current controls on innovative surgery with this one. But first a few caveats. The question of whether psychosurgery, or other innovative surgery, is "good medicine" obviously requires weighing values. If, for example, any psychosurgery has as its collateral effect marked diminution of individual capacities, then judgment about its use may turn on the significance one attaches to "capacity to reason" where preserving that capacity entails "severe depression." Value questions of this sort are present in most cases of medical intervention. Usually they are ignored because a consensus exists as to values and is so clear that the premise goes unstated. In other instances, such as whether drugs with potential for abuse should be prescribed for obesity, the value conflict is readily perceived.

Although recognition that values underlie much medical decision making is important and too often overlooked, to accomplish such recognition at the cost of losing sight of the role that data should play would be unfortunate. In most instances, wise formulation of policy is impossible without up-to-date information. The very fact that a procedure is innovative assures that the data will be filled with gaps, but incomplete data is better than no data at all if one perceives the question of whether to use an innovative procedure as subject to constant reevaluation in light of new experience. The practical problem with regard to psychosurgery in particular, and innovative surgery in general, is that the necessary information is either not collected or not made available.

What strikes the skeptical lawyer most forcefully about psychosurgery is how little information is available to persons who would undertake a review of present practices. First, no one even knows how many psychosurgical operations are performed annually, and what conditions they aim to remedy. Dr. Breggin, who went to the trouble of writing to everyone he knew of in the field, could provide only a rough estimate—400-600 annually.[14] Second, many psychosurgeons have not provided full descriptions of their diagnostic procedures, and the results thereof, which prompted surgical intervention. For example, Ronald Gass notes in Chapter 3 that a memorandum surfaced in the Detroit psychosurgery litigation indicating that Dr. Rodin, who contemplated performing psychosurgery on aggressive patients in Michigan, misunderstood Drs. Mark and Ervin's work. From reading their book,[15] Rodin was not aware that each of their patients was epileptic.[16] Third, far too little information is available concerning the outcome of the operation for the patient; most research reports are still only qualitative and at the level of providing before and after photographs. What tests are performed to measure the extent to which psychosurgery relieved the problem which led to the operation? What tests are used to measure the extent of collateral damage? Although the Michigan court in the Kaimowitz case regarded psychosurgery as a "dangerous" procedure, there is not much good evidence as to how dangerous.

I believe this is a fair report of the current situation, yet I do not intend these remarks, as an indictment of psychosurgeons.

Psychosurgery poses no issue of loose data and poor controls not also presented by far more frequently utilized surgical procedures such as, until quite recently the radical mastectomy. Indeed, progress of surgical innovations into the general repertoire of medical procedures seems more a function of a network of personal relationships than of adequate scientific appraisal. And psychosurgeons at least have as an excuse the extraordinary difficulty of measuring and ascertaining the cause of personality changes over time. Rather the fundamental problem is that there is a basic conflict between the doctor's duties as an applied scientist and duties owed to the patient who wants all the stops pulled in pursuit of therapy. The current psychosurgery situation, with the procedures in use before data necessary to evaluate them is available, stems from that dilemma.

This important conflict is an infrequently explored aspect of medical experimentation ethics. Experimentation has been commonly divided for ethical analysis into experimentation which is not undertaken to benefit the subject, and experimentation which is incident to therapy. Some ethical principles are common to both types. The first command of ethical experimentation of any kind, and the one of central importance for my purposes, is that the experiment be designed to produce useful results. The American Medical Association's Guidelines on Clinical Investigation formulates this standard:

A physician may participate in clinical investigation only to the extent that his activities are a part of a systematic program competently designed, under accepted standards of scientific research, to produce data which is scientifically valid and significant.[17]

In other aspects of the experimenter-subject relationship, particularly the extent to which consent must be "informed," the therapeutic setting has justified less rigorous rules than those pertaining to experimentation for science alone.

Formulating standards for non-therapeutic experimentation is often regarded as the critically difficult ethical problem. The philosophical issue is especially troublesome. It traps us between a utilitarian recognition that the social good obtained by carefully constructed, albeit dangerous, experiments exceeds the likely human cost, and our countervailing sense, whether it be antiutilitarian or not, that it is wrong to conscript humans as guinea pigs when there is no intention or expectation that they will benefit in any way. We escape from the cul-de-sac by a concept of "volunteering" manifested by "consent," but are then troubled by why people volunteer to expose themselves needlessly to danger. Is it because they need the money, or that they want the recognition of their professors or the consideration of their parole boards?

Therapeutic experimentation does not present these nagging questions. People likely to die next week will rationally risk a lot today; so too will those whose lives are made miserable by illness. There are still ethical issues particularly when the condition from which the experimental subject suffers may be cured by reasonably effective known techniques. Nonetheless, the basic situation is one in which we can understand and identify with the motivations of those subjects who consent. Consequently, the principal focus of ethical guidelines in such settings has been with assuring that experimentation does not corrupt the doctor-patient relationship. The patient's problems should be the physician's primary concern and not simply an excuse for performing the desired tests.

If the public policy problem is viewed not from the perspective of formulating principles, but rather securing compliance with whatever standards are adopted then non-therapeutic experimentation becomes simpler. The very absence of therapeutic intent alerts the investigator and others to the principles' applicability. Moreover, and more importantly, it is or should be obvious when no therapy is intended that risky procedures are "experiments" and should be undertaken, if at all, as part of the program of clinical investigation. An experiment that is not likely to produce useful results in terms of validating or invalidating the procedure should not be done.

If therapy is a goal, the compliance situation is more problematic. First, all medicine is "experimental" in the sense that any particular patient may prove to be an exception to the rule. In other words, providing therapy nearly always involves testing on a particular patient procedures and drugs believed to have been beneficial to others in roughly comparable circumstances. Yet the average general practitioner does not conceive himself to be a researcher under obligation to provide significant data. Nor, clearly, should he. Second, what should the physician do with a patient who cannot be helped by known techniques, but who may be helped by techniques presenting unknown risks and prospects for success? Dr. Cooper reports that he discovered an important remedy for dystonia, a crippling condition, when he accidentally cut an artery in a patient's brain.[18] Seeing the improvement in one patient, should he have done the "mistake" again, or would it have been better to set up a controlled research study to screen out any possibility of surgical placebo effects? In the absence of such controlled studies, when is the next doctor justified in trying out Dr. Cooper's mistake? Is he performing an experiment?

The important point is that no sharp dividing lines indicate which developments in medical practice are sufficiently "innovative" or "risky" that they should only be undertaken in an experimental context which respects the duty to produce significant data. The AMA's Guidelines for Clinical Investigation are therefore predicated entirely upon the physician's decision to do "clinical investigation." If the physician chooses to do "therapy" and not engage in "investigation," then the ethical duty to produce data which will permit evaluation of the procedure does not obtain. There is no anomaly in this result if the sole object is to assure that the "experimental" mentality does not destroy the doctor-patient relation. In that case, the investigator's decision to seek data is an appropriate precondition to special standards. If, however, another goal is a concern for a limiting the risks to which successive groups of patients are exposed, then the absence of standards mandating clinical investigation, not only in the Guidelines but elsewhere, is a serious problem. I believe that such a concern for risks has to be a key focus; indeed, it is largely implicit in the principle that a poorly designed experiment is unethical even if undertaken with a therapeutic purpose. It is strange to say that a poorly designed "experiment" is unethical, but that the same procedure performed without any effort to produce useful data is unobjectionable.[19]

The problem is that the needed standards cannot be devised in the form of abstract principles. Rather, the issue of when inadequately tested procedures should be put into practice is a question that can be answered only by an exceptionally close look at the seriousness of the problem sought to be addressed, the alternatives for patients if implementation is delayed, and the information available about the new procedure. No useful general principle is adequate to the task of meshing such specifics.

Two points follow, however. First, there is a need both in psychosurgery and innovative surgery generally for procedures to assure that the full range of experience with a particular technique *can* be brought to bear on the issue. How does a surgeon contemplating performing a psychosurgical procedure decide wisely whether to do so if no one knows how many other such operations have been performed, let alone with what effects? Where procedures are serious there should at least be some registry system to permit long-term follow-up of randomly selected patients. In addition, absolute confidentiality must be provided to ensure that bad results are reported fully and fairly. Finally, efforts should be made to coordinate diagnostic criteria among different investigators, or therapists, working on the same problem in order to facilitate comparisons of their data.[20]

Second, reposing in the individual doctor the sole responsibility for deciding whether to use innovative techniques is in many respects unsound. That decision must be made under the gun of seeing patients for whom the alternatives are not happy, and from whom the pressure to do *something* is strong. The burden of saying "no, we do not know enough about this yet," is a burden better shouldered collectively than left to individuals. Society does this with innovative drug therapies through FDA controls on investigational drug use. Sometimes the FDA permits new drugs to be marketed despite inadequate testing, particularly when the problem is important and the apparent advantages of the new drug are clear. A recent example was the release of L. dopa for Parkinson's disease. Frequently, however, the Agency is willing to say "sorry" until the results are in.

I shall now turn to the question of what other controls exist to regulate the process of surgical innovation of which psychosurgery is an instance.

Malpractice

This article is not the place for a comprehensive review of malpractice law.[21] The patient's opportunity to sue a doctor if injured in therapy may influence the surgeon's judgment concerning an innovative approach. But finding cases in which plaintiffs receive awards for adverse consequences of experimental therapy, in which the court decision is tied to the fact that the therapy was experimental, is difficult. This is not to say that doctors who believe themselves uniquely possessed of wisdom do not get in trouble. They occasionally do.[22] The reported case law, however, affords no basis for belief that malpractice recoveries are imposing major controls on the quality of the experimental process.

Reasons for the failure, if it be one, are not hard to find. The usual malpractice claim rests on the assertion that the doctor did his job negligently. Proof of that assertion is facilitated by plaintiff's demonstration that the unfavorable outcome he or she experienced is unusual. Most patients survive a fractured bone without amputation of a limb. There are standard ways of doing standard procedures. The point is that experience is the precursor of, and necessary to, judgments about negligence in the usual sense of that term. The essence of innovation is precisely that experience is lacking. No basis exists for saying that an innovative procedure was done carelessly simply because the patient died or got hurt. Of course, that does not end the inquiry. It may have been improper to perform the innovative operation at all. To some extent the locality rule—that doctors are held to the standards of care and use of procedures in their localities—permits decisions against physicians who try out new procedures unsuccessfully.[23] But the locality rule was primarily intended to protect doctors, had little effect on specialty practice, and is on the wane anyway. Its failure in this context is that it does not confront directly the important question of justification.

Although it is not too hard to imagine evolution of a how-many-dogs-did-you-try-it-on rule to control hasty translation of theory to practice, the central problems of therapeutic innovation, the agonizing appraisal of alternatives in circumstances in which no course of action is particularly appealing, does not lend itself easily to jury second-guessing. The problems are especially difficult since most experimenters do not work in a vacuum, but instead have colleagues with similar outlooks, at work on similar problems, who will defend their views. Finally, the difficulties of supervision by malpractice are especially acute where, as in psychosurgery, the injuries made the basis for suit may be inevitable concomitants of the procedures themselves.

There are legal routes to recovery against doctors that by-pass appraisals of medical negligence. Recently courts have put heavy pressure on the medical profession by authorizing recoveries where procedures were performed without the patient's "informed consent." The doctor has a duty to inform the patient with reasonable completeness about the risks medical procedures entail and their alternatives.[24] Although the importance of obtaining consent in the experimental context and elsewhere cannot be depreciated, such consent ought not be an alternative to other controls. No amount of informed consent removes concern that the treatments proffered to patients be likely to work.

Finally, there are other strong reasons for not relying heavily on tort litigation to control the innovative process, reasons that do not turn on the difficulties of successfully maintaining a plaintiff's case under current doctrines. First, the system adjudicates injury after the fact at the behest of an already injured party. Such a system may well tolerate too much injury before it is activated, particularly if one believes, as I do, that money damages, however generous, cannot compensate adequately for life-wrecking injuries. Second, litigation depends not only upon an injured party, but on an injured party who is willing to sue. Doctors can, and some doctors, I am told, do select their patients for innovative surgery with a veiw to whether they or their families are the sorts of people who would sue if disappointed with the procedure's outcome.

Professional Self-Regulation

A common aspect of "professions" is that such groups are responsible for disciplining their own members. The theory is that the professional deals with issues and utilizes techniques requiring special expertise, and that only those blessed with such expertise can assess his skill. The argument may be grounded more on monopoly than in reason, but it is nonetheless widely accepted in law and in medicine. The reality, however, is that professional discipline is rarely exercised in either profession.[25] Even more rarely is it brought to bear in medicine in an effort to control the quality and pacing of innovative efforts. The consequence is that no formal controls exist within the profession to supervise the process by which innovations are tried out.

The more complex psychosurgical procedures cannot be performed in the doctor's office, and therefore the doctor who wishes to do them must have access to a hospital. But few formal controls exist at the hospital level either. That remains true despite the strengthening of requirements that funded research be subjected to peer group review as a precondition to obtaining federal grants.[26] Those institutional review committees are charged, of course, with weighing the hard questions of whether patients in experiments, regardless of therapeutic purpose, are being exposed to inappropriate risks. But to date, such institutional screening has been made mandatory only in instances where people perceive that they are researching. Thus, this useful development does not resolve the hard problem: What procedures should be undertaken only as a part of a research project designed to develop evidence concerning their efficacy? Very few hospitals have committees whose express responsibility is to assess the right to perform proposed operations, and with what frequency and evaluation. The absence of such formal committee oversight is especially troublesome in as much as most innovations in surgery do not occur in the course of externally funded research, and thus will never be reviewed by experimentation committees.

I do not know why hospitals have not established such oversight. It may reflect both tradition and law. Usually the hospital is not legally responsible for the torts of doctors who exercise operating privileges.[27] The patient deals with the surgeon, and the hospital provides services. Hospitals have fought to maintain the rule that they are not responsible for every doctor's mistakes. Yet if the hospital gets into the business of approving innovative procedures, it may well become legally responsible for mishaps, a responsibility that probably could not be disclaimed.[28] This concern for possible liability may have led hospital administrators to steer clear of extensive oversight of innovation, and one can easily understand why they might be cautious. In other words, the situation may be one, all too frequent in our society, in which rules of law have a completely unintended impact on the way people behave.

In any event, I believe that expanded committee review to encompass whether procedures should be regarded as innovative, and setting ground rules for their evaluation, would be highly desirable. On one front, of course, such committees may check hasty efforts which the practitioner might characterize as the search for a dramatic leap. Equally important, however, such committee oversight, by facilitating evaluation and adding credibility to reported results, might encourage more rapid adoption of advances which do work.

Two observations about formal committee review should be emphasized. First, it cannot be regarded as a panacea. Anyone who has served on committees of any sort will recognize that proponents of measures (when they know more about the problem, care more about the committee's action, and have done their homework) are well situated to secure favorable committee action on proposals which, in retrospect and with more work, seem patently foolish. This reality of human nature is not likely to yield to any tinkering with organizational flow charts in medicine or elsewhere. But that committees will be of limited effect does not imply that they are useless. Indeed, simply requiring the surgeon to realize that "innovation" is going on, and to reflect on how it may be evaluated, may be a large step in the right direction.

Second, I have stressed formal oversight. Surely there exist very powerful controls in hospitals that are not formalized. Raised eyebrows at lunch or fear of being thought a charlatan can be powerful restraints on inappropriate conduct—indeed, they may be just as potent as formal regulation. Nonetheless, examining the history of psychosurgery as told by Dr. Vaughan in Chapter 2 shows numerous instances of procedures being done in circumstances where the necessity of making a formal presentation to an interdisciplinary group would likely have called a halt to the trials.

132

Federal Regulatory Controls: The Drug/Surgery Contrast

Psychosurgery has developed without any systematic oversight by public agencies charged with collecting, evaluating, or approving new developments. This does not mean that the government has not sponsored conferences and review efforts, for it has. But the general approach has been ad hoc. Once again, however, pointing the finger at psychosurgery and its practitioners would be completely misleading, for the same ad hoc approach characterizes most government efforts in reviewing innovative surgery—a point that was well demonstrated when the heart transplant operation burst upon the scene. The ad hoc approach results from our entrusting to the profession the responsibility for its own assessment and self-discipline.

In this section I wish briefly to make a point well worth an independent research project. Although I do not advocate tight federal controls over surgery, there are differences between our regulatory approaches to drugs and to surgery which may well have extremely pernicious consequences, especially in therapeutic settings where drugs and surgical procedures are likely to be alternatives. (Psychosurgery is surely such a setting; performing circumcision is surely not.) Making the point requires a brief overview of the legal requirements for marketing new drugs.

"New drugs" may not be "introduced" into interstate commerce without approval by the FDA. Securing such approval for general marketing is a complex process, and only the main points need be mentioned. Essentially, the manufacturer must show both that the drug is safe and, by "substantial evidence," that it is effective. Substantial evidence is interpreted to require controlled clinical trials. For the purpose of investigating the drug to ascertain whether it is safe and effective, the Secretary is directed to promulgate regulations authorizing use of the drug for investigational purposes by qualified experts, thus giving limited exemption from the otherwise applicable restraint on "introducing." Before such exemption is given, adequate preclinical tests must be done. Moreover, the sponsors of human research must agree to keep such records as may be required in the course of experimentation on humans to facilitate the ultimate determination of effectiveness called for by statute. Finally, the statute and

133

regulations set forth rather detailed standards requiring that persons used as investigational subjects give their informed consent in all but a few instances.

Even after the drug is approved for general marketing, the control process continues. The product must be labeled to provide adequate directions and warnings concerning its use. The FDA also regulates product advertising. Finally, the manufacturer is obligated to keep records to facilitate prompt recognition of new hazards found to be associated with the drug. Independently, a nationally organized system of reporting hospitals and physicians monitors adverse drug reactions.[29]

Many have claimed that these protections are less than meet the eye, and several instances of flagrant evasion of responsibility by drug manufacturers have surfaced.[30] Nonetheless, the drug law represents a national commitment to keep compounds off the market until they are well studied. But this commitment is not without cost. Some people die or stay sick because drugs that would have helped are not yet generally available; moreover, the pace of innovation is surely affected by the manufacturers' recognition of the cost of the process of securing approval, which means that drugs that might have been discovered have not been. Indeed, the case could be argued that the number of drug accidents prevented by FDA controls is far fewer than the number of patients who suffer needlessly because innovation is so hampered. Whatever the truth of this assertion, the FDA approval process plainly entails a balance of risks.[31]

The contrast between controls the FDA imposes and those existing on innovative surgery is stark. Surgical innovations which inevitably cause severe discomfort, and many of which are very dangerous, proceed from innovative stages to general use without any comprehensive regulatory effort to assess their safety and effectiveness. If "psychosurgery" were a pill, it could not conceivably be marketed at this time.

There are differences between surgery and drug therapies which would make simple-minded extension of federal controls ludicrous. I shall discuss them in a moment. It does seem worth emphasizing, however, that prima facie it is wrong to draw the "benefit-risk" balance at different places for probably interchangeable therapies, and this surely is the situation now, in that surgical risks are tolerated where chemical ones would not be. For example, to deny patients access to a drug causing severe adverse reactions in .01 percent of all cases, when the consequence is that the patient undergoes surgery with a .02 percent chance of killing him to accomplish the same cure, is silly.

No one contemplating this dilemma, however, should fail to note its complexities. Surgical procedures are fully under "professional" control and are thus protected by the tradition of a profession as a self-regulating group. The formal subjects of regulation by the FDA are manufacturers, not practicing doctors. The distinction is important for several reasons. First, the surgeon rests the decision to employ innovative surgery on personal experience and on the information given by colleagues. By contrast, the doctor using new drugs has to rely initially on evidence assembled by the drug companies. These companies undoubtedly have a moral duty, as well as some economic interest, in truth telling. But they are also subject to conflicting pressure to maximize current profits by fostering the widest possible use of their products. The need of some regulation of the claims they make to achieve this result is, I believe, self-evident.

Indication of the current importance of professional control as a justification for nonregulation may be gained by considering how few are the legal restraints on the uses doctors make of new drugs once they come onto the market. Prescribing the drugs at levels far in excess of those officially ascertained by the FDA to be safe and effective is not a crime. Quite the contrary, the medical community's practice is to regard the manufacturer's brochures as too conservative, and to rely instead on the gradual accumulation of collegial wisdom in using higher dosages. In a well-known malpractice case, *Salgo* v. *Leland Stanford, Jr., University Board of Trustees* experts testified that "local practice" had crystallized and called for administration of the drug Urokon in more than twice the manufacturer's recommended dosage when performing translumbar aortagraphy.[32]

Second, surgery has no analogue to the drug manufacturer, upon whom may be placed the burden of systematic monitoring of experience. The current FDA controls are so expensive to comply with that only the prospect of high profits induces the effort. Comparable returns are not possible for the innovative surgeon, even were it possible to organize the documentation without which FDA review would be ineffective.[33] Moreover, augmenting the problem is a difference in standardization. With drugs one is dealing with a "thing," the characteristics of which can be tested in a variety of ways. Although it is true that apparently identical chemical substances turn out to behave rather differently, and that different doctors get strikingly different results testing the "same" drug, the fact remains that to a far greater extent the safety and effectiveness of surgical procedures depends on who is doing them.

These considerations obviously militate against any heavy-handed control of innovative surgery. But the issue is whether the public health hazards posed by these alternative therapeutic techniques, surgery and drugs, are so different that we can be comfortable with the informal control situation as it exists to-day. I think not. I am not now ready, however, to offer much by way of an alternative, other than to stress the points made earlier about collection of data and coordination of research.

It may seem strange in a chapter devoted to psychosurgery to stress so heavily at the outset general considerations which pertain to most innovative surgery. Nonetheless, the guts of the psycho-surgery problem is that there is too little trustworthy information despite the surgeons' having performed a considerable number of operations. Moreover, realization that this failure has as much to do with the fact that surgery is involved as that the surgery is "psycho"—a consideration relevant in this context only because it complicates measurement—has important policy implications.

Many proposals for restraining psychosurgery, proposals which are defended because good data about psychosurgery are lacking, seek to isolate psychosurgery by imposing special public oversight requirements. The Oregon legislation creates a "psychosurgery board" having the duty, among others, of deciding "whether or not the operation has clinical merit and is an appropriate treat-ment for the specific patient."[34] In reaching this finding the review board may consult the literature and consult with experts to assess whether the operation has "clinical merit." In addition, to warrant a decision that the operation is appropriate for the patient, the board must find, *inter alia*, that "all conventional therapies have been exhausted" and that "all other viable alternative methods of treatment have been tried and have failed to produce satisfactory results."

I have some reservations about this sort of legislation simply because the legislative process does not respond quickly enough to changed circumstances. For example, if some psychosurgery is shown to be effective and safer than drugs, I believe it is foolish to require conventional therapy first.[35] Yet I doubt that the legislation will be quickly rewritten. More importantly, however, the premise of the legislation is wrong. The assumption is that psychosurgery is unique in the extent to which very serious procedures are performed with inadequate understanding of what will happen. As the prior discussion of innovative surgery indicates, I doubt this very much. Thus while I have no objection to public oversight of medicine, the use of comparable resources for review in any number of other areas may advance the public's safety and welfare much further. Isolating psychosurgery simply masks the deeper problems.

To be sure, objections and fears about psychosurgery are not predicated only upon inadequate data. Tampering so grossly with a person's brain raises philosophical problems about human identity. Moreover, the capacity to change people dramatically without acting through their sensory processes raises fears of political repression or medical tyranny. Three observations about these issues are appropriate by way of introduction to the problems of consent discussed in the next section.

First, psychosurgery is hardly likely to be a major instrument of political repression. The techniques necessary to do the modern procedures are so refined, and the equipment so expensive, that all the neurosurgeons in the country working around the clock would make little dent on the population at large. By contrast, drugs are cheap to manufacture and little skill is needed to require their ingestion. Routine administration of chloropromazine at mental institutions around the country is a far more serious political problem than psychosurgery.[36] Moreover, sophisticated use of ancient principles of psychology is probably more potent than either "medical" technique in influencing the way masses of people behave.

Second, if psychosurgery does "work," by which I mean that in the judgment of the medical profession it relieves a patient's problems without inappropriate risks, then I see no adequate reason to prohibit it when the patient wants it done. The burden of such a denial falls most heavily on the patient, and strong reasons must be found to justify overriding his wishes.

Third, psychosurgery and other behavior control techniques raise especially serious fears of medical overreaching in cases where consent is by proxy, or where the patient's consent is inevitably influenced by the prospect of evading social restraint. There is no way, however, of protecting fully against such overreaching without adopting rules so restrictive that their cost in suffering exceeds their worth. As a practical matter, the single most important protection available for such patients is the assurance that proferred treatments are likely to work—a pledge we have not honored in the past.

Consent and Autonomy

The Competent Adult

Discussing whether the community should prohibit outright or drastically limit by law the performance of psychosurgical procedures is a complex task. For me there are a variety of possible answers, each of which turns upon premises which may or may not be accurate, or which may be accurate now but invalid five years from now. I find it helpful to start with two simplifying assumptions. I shall assume both that the medical community believes on the basis of adequate scientific evidence that psychosurgery "works," in that its benefits are greater than its risks, and that a competent adult requests that such a procedure be done.

Whether Consent Should Be Allowed. The contention that society should reject completely the use of psychosurgical procedures regardless of what doctors as a group think about them must, I think, rest on one or more of three propositions. First, the conditions sought to be treated are not "medical problems"; second, medicine should not interfere, or at least not interfere irreversibly, with the "executive apparatus" of the person—the mental processes controlling "willing," "feeling," and other aspects of the private self; or third, that the possible side effects of psychosurgery are so severe in terms of an individual's "human-ness" that they may not be inflicted for any reason. The first two arguments do not convince me once the assumptions of this discussion are granted: The professionals (operating under better controls) ascertain that the procedures on balance provide better results than other therapies might do, and the patient concurs in the decision to have the operation performed. As to the third, I believe the factual predicate is lacking.

Medical Problems. There are real difficulties in defining in fixed fashion what conditions may properly be called "medical prob-lems." Thus far the law has rarely done so for purposes of limiting the powers of licensed physicians. Rather medical problems are those unwanted conditions doctors as a group purport to have the ability to treat. Limits that have been imposed on individual doctors in treating consenting patients usually reflect application of supposed medical expertise to a particular mode of treatment. Thus, although maiming is a crime even where done with consent, if enough doctors regard the penectomy (sex change) operation as sound medical practice for treating psychological problems inci-dent to confirmed transsexuality, it is not criminal maiming. If only one doctor thought so, that doctor might be in trouble. Similarly, enforcement or threatened enforcement of the narcotics laws against doctors who insisted on regarding addiction as a medical problem to be treated by, or in conjunction with, maintenance doses of narcotics was done in the name of "good medical practice." There are some instances, but not many, in which the medical community's judgment is of minor importance. For example, the medical profession's views concerning abortion as appropriate therapy for unwanted pregnancy does not vitiate objection to abortion in some states. On the whole, the practice of letting the profession find its limits is sound, and reflects the belief that the public should not interfere with the individual's choice when what he or she wants or is willing to have done is supported by competent medical assessment that it is appropriate. By permitting consent, the patient's autonomy is preserved.

One potentially troublesome consequence of allowing "medical conditions" to be delimited by professional assessment of what can be treated effectively is that the number of such conditions grows along with the wonders of the physician's armamentarium. Medical aid is not limited to clear concepts of disease and injury—fighting germs and mending bones. Rather doctors become producers of effects. They can wake you up, put you to sleep, and in between keep you pleasured but childless. This process of medical expansion creates risks with which public policy must be concerned although the treatments are proferred only to those whose legally effective consent has been secured. The first is the problem of stigmatization.

By stigmatization I mean that socially understood concepts of disease and injury grow to encompass conditions that doctors have the power to change. Chronic sadness becomes a disease when drugs are available to treat it. Such redefinition does not always happen. Most people do not regard a lined face as a disease simply because a facelift will "cure" it. Redefinition does occur, however, in situations in which producing the effect will minimize social tensions, particularly when responsibility for producing the tension is in doubt. If you and I don't get along, and doing nothing about it is intolerable for a variety of reasons, the options are that you change, I change, or we do not associate (an option that also is often intolerable). That the doctors can change you and not me suggests that you are the one to change. Thus if high-strung children and boring schools do not mix, and schools cannot be made less boring but must be attended, tranquilize the children. It makes sense to intervene where you can. But people do not like to accept or even think about their responsibility in such situations, particularly if they might change but do not want to change. Stigmatization helps in the process. That the doctor, the same person who kills viruses and mends broken legs, *can* change you indicates that you are "sick" and I am "healthy." Whatever my moral responsibility for making you sick, you are the one to undergo treatment. Moreover, your being sick limits your responsibility. You are not responsible for being sick, but you are responsible for burdening me with a disease you might easily cure.

This process of stigmatization by labeling poses serious risks when, as I shall soon discuss, "proxy" consent is involved. The "I" in the situation described has authority to ascertain what is good for the "you." It also makes one question ordinary garden variety consent. The risk is that the consenting individual has internalized the labels unthinkingly and does not "really" understand the situation, especially when the people around him are calling him sick and asking why he does not do something about it. For example, Dr. Delgado recounted at the Hastings Institute Conference on Physical Brain Manipulation that a girl had seen him seeking ESB. She hoped that this novel technique might cure her of her propensity to behave so flirtatiously that she provoked fights in bars. Was she upset because of involvement in fights and with the police, or was she upset because other people acted as though she were sick?

There are no easy solutions to this old problem of the tyranny of labels, a problem that has no new dimension just because psychosurgery is in the picture. One possibility, however, is to say that the validity and appropriateness of individual consent are so doubtful that the remedy ought be prohibited. Whether physical manipulation of the brain (PMB) alters behavior with acceptable risks is irrelevant if it is morally repugnant to give credence to any patient's request that we do it. I believe it would be monstrous to be so reluctant. To ignore the patient understates the awareness that people can have about themselves. Moreover, it minimizes the seriousness of the conditions that the patient may be left to handle. There are frame-of-reference problems here as well, as most authors on these subjects do not have to live with the patient's condition. Finally, the consequence of barring psychosurgery if it works is to remit people to therapies which by hypothesis do not work as well, when "consent" on the theory outlined ought to be equally ineffective. We have gone too far down the road charted by Freud to think that serious personality disorders will escape the labeling process or be denied treatment, however ineffective.

Another danger posed by the expansion of "medical conditions" concerns situations in which wide-scale employment of a medically produced effect, even assuming it works, is safe, and that consent is fully "informed," has serious consequences for the social order. The risk is that such issues will be left to doctors on the assumption that only another facet of medicine is involved. For example, suppose science develops, as is likely, simple techniques to provide parental choice of the sex of their unconceived children. The issue of whether and when such techniques should be made available in the face of evidence that they could have massive impact on population structure is so far removed from the normal ambit of medical decision making that it would be strange to assign doctors primary competence for setting the standards. Similarly, there may be problems when medical techniques alter the parameters of human potential. If "performance" drugs improving intelligence are marketed widely, everyone is subject to pressure to use them so as not to be left behind in our intelligence centered society.

Psychosurgery does not pose issues of this character. No one is likely to be so treated unless he or she is perceived as abnormal. But in any event, I believe the only response to such issues is to consider each technique on its merits. That we will blindly leave to doctors whether brain implantation is to be generally used in service of education is, I think, an unlikely prospect. The very fact that a procedure is used throughout the population undercuts the focus on "abnormality" that gives the labeling process such force, particularly when the social disruption feared has no particular medical significance.

Acting Irreversibly on the Brain. Assuming that there is nothing untoward in doctors treating the sort of behavioral and personality disorders that prompt psychosurgery, is there any special significance in the fact that these procedures act directly and irreversibly on the brain? In the case of a consenting patient, I think not. First, there cannot be an objection to operating on the brain as such; no one would countenance denying surgical relief to those with tumors. For the same reason, I do not believe any effort to ascribe central significance to particular brain sites on the grounds that they are the center of the personality can be successful. Most of us would not hold to such views in the face of evidence that a person's aberrant behavior resulted from a tumor located dead center in whatever brain matter is thought to be the repository of the "will."

Is it relevant for setting regulatory policy that the patient has no tumor or other evidence of brain pathology, and that doctors are operating simply because of behavior? Where short-term effects on personality are involved, I see no issues not also present by prescription of psychoactive drugs. Therefore, I believe the only serious problem is whether a person should be allowed to consent to permanent destruction of part of the brain if no medical showing can be made that anything is wrong with it other than that it "produces" unwanted behavior. That is the situation as regards some psychosurgery. But why should one care whether the patient's brain is damaged? The criterion that organic abnormality must precede treatment is not followed generally, either in psychiatry or general medicine.[37]

In thinking about this problem, three of its aspects should be distinguished. First, demonstration of brain pathology may be one technique for demonstrating that performance of an operation is "good medicine." The fact that one can say that (a) the patient's brain is damaged in a particular way, (b) most people who have such damage behave aberrantly as does the patient, and (c) this operation has worked to change that behavior in other patients, goes far to alleviate the fears of some critics that psychosurgeons are cutting without much understanding of where and what they cut. Utilization of evidence of pathology for this purpose is simply another way of talking about the profession's efforts, publicly regulated or not, to assure that what they do "works" while creating predictable and limited risks. Whether brain pathology is important in this sense is just another issue of quality control. It may be an immensely important practical issue, but no matter of independent moral significance is involved.

Second, evidence of brain damage or disease may be a limited but useful regulatory device to control coercive or quasi-coercive uses of these psychosurgical techniques, depending upon one's views about the extent to which "pathology" is itself a concept with real content. Thus, one possible check on using psychosurgery to control nonconformity is that parents, spouses, or the state may not authorize that procedures be done to control behavior or emotions which are "aberrant," but to which no underlying pathology can be shown. A distant analogue to such a requirement is the principle, found in the *Model Penal Code*'s test of criminal responsibility, that one may not infer mental disease or defect from an abnormality manifested only by repeated instances of criminal or antisocial conduct.[38] Whether a comparable limitation on psychosurgery makes sense depends on what one means by pathology. For example, suppose that nearly all excessively violent people can be shown by increasingly sensitive monitoring equipment to have EEG patterns that differ from the patterns of nonaggressive people. Does that constitute evidence of pathology? Is pathology shown if these patterns are related directly to measurable differences in certain brain sites? If "yes" is the answer to either question, then pathology may well be a delusion, and the only question is how long it takes for researchers to show that pathology is another way of talking about aberrant behavior. On the other hand, if pathology is not shown by demonstrated brain "abnormality" on a cellular level correlated directly with aberrant behavior, what does one mean by brain pathology? Is the concept limited to damage produced by "accidents" like childhood beatings?

The third and broadest use of evidence of brain pathology would be to limit the use of brain intervention procedures even on consenting adults where no such limitation is suggested by medical considerations alone. The advantage of such a rule is that, assuming that brain pathology is a meaningful concept, it mitigates some of the fears expressed earlier concerning the quality of individual consent. The individual's consent to be operated upon cannot be given effect if all that supports it are the labels that pass for analysis of mental illness. By contrast, if pathology is shown, there is less need to worry about overreaching.

On balance, I do not think that imposition of a "pathology" limitation regarding consenting patients would be wise. My reasons are a mixture of doubts about the "pathology" concept coupled with a strong preference for allowing people to have what they want when there are not strong grounds for denying it. Certainly authorizing a doctor to destroy part of one's brain is a grim and serious task. But we usually allow people to make serious decisions about themselves, including decisions which will have long-lasting consequences. Therefore, I would rather focus on creating better mechanisms to improve a patient's understanding of the consequences of the changes, than have doctors say "no" to a patient because they cannot find the requisite evidence of impairment. Let me make clear the hypothesis, however: The doctors find that pathology has no significance either in terms of benefits and risks of the procedure itself, or in terms of the likelihood that other, less drastic procedures may be successful. Whether that hypothesis is accurate is a matter I am not competent to judge.

Seriousness of Side Effects. The third problem of accepting consent concerns the issue of seriousness of side effects. We do not allow people suffering from mental problems to commit suicide.[39] At what point does destruction of an individual's intelligence, judgment, and so on, become so dehumanizing that we ought not allow it, even though the body that remains reports itself happy? In theory the issue is appropriate for community rule making which overrides individual consent. Whether such regulation makes sense as a practical matter, however, depends on whether the collateral effects of psychosurgery as presently practiced are sufficiently severe to raise serious risks of this sort. As I understand the situation, the risks are not this serious, but the absence of reliable evidence has already been noted.

Ascertaining Appropriate Consent. Thus far, the discussion has been based upon simplifying assumptions, particularly that the medical community regards the procedures as effective. It is now time to explore some complications. First, many might deny that the medical community should be the judge of efficacy; second, no consensus as to efficacy currently exists; third, in the present situation there are grounds for concern about the quality of consent.

My preference for leaving the judgment about efficacy to the medical profession is based entirely upon practical considerations. In our society most decisions about medical intervention are made pursuant to the so-called medical model. Professionals assess the possible benefits and harms the particular patient may experience as a consequence of intervention. The decision to intervene requires not only legally effective consent by or for the patient, but also a judgment by the professionals that such consent is appropriate.

Appropriateness is the central problem because it calls for balancing benefits and risks. Appropriateness is, of course, a concept loaded with values. Often the benefits medical intervention may product cannot be assessed against their risks except by value judgments that relate two incommeasurables. That is particularly the case when surgery destroys one body function to save another. For example, consider the issue of what risks to life justify amputation of a limb, or whether it is appropriate to blind children intentionally in order to prevent the spread of a tumor which might or might not spread if left untreated, but will kill them if it does spread. Such questions are "medical" issues in a special sense. Medicine is the context in which they arise, and that profession has a tradition of worrying about them. But their resolution plainly turns not on specialized medical knowledge but rather on how one values life itself as against its various components, a matter on which doctors have no pipeline to truth. Nonetheless, society usually leaves such problems to the self-regulation of the medical community. The justification is that the decisions reached by the profession are not sufficiently different from those society would reach to warrant the difficulties, inconvenience, and expense of community oversight.

The regulatory question that concerns psychosurgery and other PMB therapies is whether the issue of appropriateness of use in this special area should be left to the medical community as have other treatment decisions. The argument against so doing is by and large the same as that presented earlier concerning "medical conditions." Doctors have no special claim to expertise about whether provocative promiscuity is better left "untreated" than "cured" at the cost of substantial diminution of other human capacities. The trouble with that argument, however, is that it encompasses far too much. Doctors qua doctors are equally "incompetent" to judge the other value issues with which they are routinely presented. The important point bears repetition: The justification for confiding such issues to doctors is not that they are somehow qualified by training and expertise to decide them, but rather that we do not think the probability that we would decide them differently warrants the effort of self-education.

Therefore, the public policy arguments for moving from the medical model should not be couched in terms of whether the involvement is "behavior" rather than "disease." The real issue is whether we believe that the medical community on the whole has a value system with respect to the matter in dispute which is sufficiently different from the community's to make societal intervention appropriate. For example, in regard to prolonging life, I believe such a discrepancy does exist. Doctors' whole professional experience is so wrapped up in life saving that they are too commonly unwilling to let the terminally ill patient go comfortably, quickly, and cheaply. But I see no reason to think that doctors as a group are disposed to regard trivial behavioral conditions as warranting partial brain destruction, or that they balance behavioral manifestations versus risks of treatment in any unusual way. That is particularly the case in as much as good doctors treat the "patient" anyway. Disease is relevant only because of the impact it has on the patient's life.

Thus I see no compelling reason to suggest that evaluation of the balancing entailed by psychosurgery be done by nonphysicians. To be sure, adding laymen to a psychosurgery board, will not hurt, and may well be justified simply as a means of inspiring public confidence. In my brief experience, however, doctors are so much more sophisticated about the facts, risks, benefits, and alternatives which may develop in the near future that no one should be surprised if their judgment dominates any such group.

Confidence in the consensus of medical opinion and confidence in individual doctors are two different things, however. We do not now have any general medical consensus about the relative efficacy of psychosurgery in treating the variety of conditions for which it has been used. Because of inadequate attention to the data-gathering process and the necessity of evaluation, there is little upon which such a consensus can rest.

There are, I believe, only three broad regulatory options now open. We may prohibit psychosurgery entirely or dramatically limit by law the conditions for which such procedures may be employed. I think such a course is foolish unless it is believed either that such treatments are never going to be of any significant

147

medical use, or that their utility can be ascertained by processes which do not entail their use.

Alternatively, we can do nothing, and leave the regulatory situation alone. That course is equally unsatisfactory. Granted that psychosurgery may not be so different from other surgery in the extent to which it has grown without adequate evaluation. Nonetheless, the procedures may interfere irreversibly with basic aspects of personality, and they are commonly done on patients whose level of comprehension is especially suspect.

I believe a middle course should be charted. Until such time as adequate understanding of the procedures is developed, I believe they should be utilized only in accord with special controls, at the heart of which should be the principle of multispecialty patient diagnosis and evaluation, and especially sensitive attention to assuring informed consent. Such controls might be instituted either through legislation or through professional self-regulatory efforts. Between the two I currently favor professional self-regulation.

The significant advantage of legislative treatment of psychosurgery is that uniform rules can be imposed over a wide geographic area either directly or, more probably, through a commission. There is less fear that professional standards will be evaded by gravitation of dubious work to dubious institutions. But the price paid for that advantage is also significant. First, as I indicated earlier in discussing the problem of evaluation, psychosurgery is a dramatized instance of a set of problems. To focus legislative attention on it alone invites a splintered approach to problems that demand unified effort. The likely consequence of a psychosurgery board is an unhelpful polarization of the situation. The parties in interest become the psychosurgeon and a board, with the rest of the profession taking the view that the problem is not theirs. Moreover, there will be a tendency for the success of any such board to be measured only by the outcome of operations it allows. There are real disadvantages in creating institutions which are publicly accountable only along one dimension of complex issues. Parole boards are perceived to fail when they release offenders who turn out to be dangerous; incarcerating the reformable to the point that they are ruined is not something for which parole boards will be widely damned. Similarly, the FDA rightly wants to avoid recurrence of the thalidomide tragedy, for such regulatory failures will be laid at its door. But it is not keelhauled in the press because in an excess of caution patients suffer age-old infirmities that might have been averted by more daring therapies.

Second, legislation is often counterproductive in highly fluid situations, particularly legislation which mandates compliance with complex rules before action can be taken. An example is provided by the Oregon legislation requiring that all conventional therapy be used before psychosurgery is employed. One can imagine evidence developing which would make that rule grossly unfair to patients. Yet once on the books, the rule must be obeyed until amended.

Given these problems with the legislative board approach, I favor more limited regulatory remedies for patients who are competent to consent. The most important have been discussed: recognition that the procedures are experimental, establishment of registries, and multispecialty diagnosis and evaluation under professionally devised guidelines. If further protection from abuse is thought necessary, then I would prefer to control it by prohibiting the procedures except when done in certain research facilities, facilities that could then be controlled through the funding process. Such an approach is practical, given the infrequency with which psychosurgery is performed.

Proxy Consent

The most difficult issues concerning psychosurgery and other therapies involving PMB are the propriety of their use in circumstances in which the patient is not competent to consent to their use. There are a variety of reasons why the patient may be incompetent, and each of them might be made subject to different rules. For example, the patient may be a child and thus lack capacity to give any effective consent. The patient may be legally competent, but nonetheless sufficiently deranged or dull witted so that purported consent would lack credence. This situation is likely to be present and be especially complex if the patient has been committed, voluntarily or involuntarily, to a mental institution to receive treatment. Or the patient may have been found incompetent in proceedings leading to the appointment of a guardian.

The law usually responds to the dilemma of a person who cannot say yes or no by allowing others to act in the person's interests—sometimes subject to judicial oversight, as with guardians. For example, parents may authorize the doctors to perform a tonsilectomy on a child; the child's wishes may be irrelevant.[40] A spouse may authorize a doctor to perform an operation on an elderly patient who has become unconscious. Similarly, doctors are permitted to treat a patient in a mental institution on the theory that treatment is in the patient's interests, and were the patient to understand the situation he would consent. In its choice of representatives the law operates in part on a fiction: that parents, spouses, and public doctors have the best interests of the patient in mind because their concerns are congruent. Plainly, that need not be the case, as parents often enough hate their children, and spouses one another. But for most purposes the rules work well enough, especially since the decision to have any treatment whatever rests upon the medical model described earlier. The doctor must decide that consent to the risks entailed is appropriate. Operations are not bought in the supermarket. Moreover, no alternatives to the rule of representation are feasible or desirable regarding the majority of issues. Most people would be outraged if major decisions concerning the health of their children were taken from their hands. If we distrust families, we trust indifferent bureaucracies even less.

Psychosurgery, however, poses very special problems for reasons touched upon earlier. Mental illness, violent behavior, and the other conditions for which such procedures have been touted involve complex relationships between the person and his or her environment. For example, in the case of the supposedly promiscuous girl, it is impossible to be sure wherein the problem lies, for without the social stigma attached to such behavior there would be no occasion for therapy. Moreover, the behavior may not be upsetting to the patient but only to the people with whom she deals, who are precisely those to whom the law commonly looks for consent. One incident recounted at a conference on psychosurgery illustrates the problem.[41] A man in a fit of violent rage tried unsuccessfully to hit his wife with a cleaver. Subsequently, whether to perform a psychosurgical procedure became an issue. Should we look to his wife as the proper person to give consent if he cannot comprehend? They share a community of interest, but to expect her to weigh the decision without regard to her own fears asks too much. Certainly concern for the quality of her decision-making process can be overstated. Some restraint is, or ought to be, imposed because the judgment must be made by the surgeon that the operation is on balance a worthwhile effort. The response that surgeons are sloppy or too eager to do their experiments suggests the need for broader reforms, not special rules directed only at proxy consent.

Despite the general protections of the medical model, the setting tends to prompt questionable action. The physician almost inevitably becomes a double agent with loyalties not to the patient alone but to the full set of participants with whom he or she must deal. In Chapter 2 Dr. Vaughan provides an interesting example of how Japanese psychosurgeons have acted in response to their culture's strong disapproval of institutionalizing children, no matter how unmanageable. In deciding to operate the surgeons are thus weighing in the balance factors such as the parents' disgrace which may not be important to the patient.

The double-agent problem is by no means the only one. Even more troublesome is that our perceptions about what is or is not desirable are structured by our culture-bound frames of reference. If I see someone obviously suffering intense emotional pain, my immediate response is that he would be better off changed. If the person so afflicted says "I like it this way," I am even more convinced that he is very sick. These are familiar, albeit poorly resolved, dilemmas of both law and psychiatry. Although there is considerable force to the argument that the patient's wishes should be honored, what should be done when the patient can say nothing which would indicate that "his" views are entitled to respect? The temptation, given our bias toward normalcy, is to say that since I would want treatment, he should want treatment. There is perhaps no great objection to so doing in most cases, but where irreversible destruction of capacities is concerned, as in psychosurgery, I believe we are obliged to give the matter closer attention.

Finally, these problems achieve their most complex dimension when the physician's double-agent status and culture-bound values act upon a patient whose alternatives are socially restricted. For example, consider a patient for whom the alternative to a psychosurgical procedure is indefinite confinement in the back ward of a mental institution, with the inevitable debilitation of such confinement. Is that prospect, which may be imposed to protect society, relevant in assessing whether psychosurgery should be done? To say it is not may doom people to unnecessary misery of extended duration, but to permit the operation may make drastic therapy more a function of legislative funding levels for mental illness than of anything peculiar to the patient.

Seeing these dilemmas is far easier than blazing a trail for their resolution. What is too little understood is that there are only a limited number of things that can be done. Moreover, like many ethical issues, their acceptable resolution turns upon unavailable facts which might easily push the balance in any direction. Whether we should allow psychosurgery to be performed upon children, given the present absence of data about the relative efficacy of such procedures in adults, is one question. Whether we should allow such procedures to be performed as part of an experimental project if efficacy in adults is shown is another. Whether there should be special rules about children no matter what the evidence shows is still a third problem. To toss solutions out without making plain one's premises about the evidence is ill advised.

My own views concerning regulation stem largely from the circumstance that the state of the evidence concerning psychosurgery is in considerable doubt. Moreover, we do not have the necessary structures to ensure that current operations will be done only after appropriately full diagnosis, psychiatric and neurological, with an intention to evaluate the procedure fully. Unless and until such structures are established, or the evidence is otherwise clarified, a moratorium should be declared upon use of psychosurgery on patients who cannot give full consent themselves. Such a proposal finds considerable support in the recent Detroit psychosurgery case, described in Chapter 3.[42] The central thrust of the Court's opinion is that we know too little about these procedures to permit them to be done on these people now. The Michigan decision does not apply to all psychosurgery, but only to that done on involuntarily committed patients. Moreover, the particular procedure was designed to remedy aggressive behavior; perhaps the judges' skepticism would have been less had the procedure been proposed as a remedy for serious depression not amenable to drug therapies. Nonetheless, I believe those possible variations should have no effect on the outcome. In the absence of far better controls than now exist, we would do well to be chary of trying innovative therapies with such potentially serious consequences on persons whose susceptibility to manipulation for others' purposes is so great.

This is not an endorsement of the Kaimowitz opinion. Leaving aside whether the case was not moot because the doctor did not wish to operate and the patient had withdrawn his consent, the court's reasoning was unsound. Thus the court emphasized that institutionalization necessarily vitiates consent. Yet the arguments the court accepted on the point would render impermissible an institutionalized patient's consent to anything, a result the court did not want and dismissed by fiat. Consent to "accepted neurological procedures" will continue to be adequate despite the "inherent coercion" and "dependency" of life within an institution.[43] More puzzling, the court framed the issue before it to include not only whether a patient might consent, but also whether a guardian might consent for him. Since it was answered that consent may not be given, guardians presumably may not consent to psychosurgery in Wayne County, Michigan. But not a word was said by the court in explanation. Surely the guardian is not reduced to dependency because the patient is hospitalized, and if the fear is that the guardian will be a malleable spouse or parent, other alternatives might be found.

I also doubt whether much is to be gained by treating psychosurgery as a First Amendment issue as the opinion does. The theory advanced by the court is that "impairing the power to generate ideas inhibits the full dissemination of ideas,"[44] thus making free speech standards relevant in appraising psychosurgery.

The proposition is not discriminating enough. Some people are so disturbed that they cannot think, and depriving them of an operation may reduce their potential to generate ideas. Moreover, independently of whether psychosurgery may facilitate "idea generation," the decision whether one wishes to generate ideas, and of what sort, would itself seem entitled to First Amendment protection on the court's theory. One can be concerned about consent, but if the First Amendment is relevant, it provides as forceful reasons for accepting the patient's "I consent" as for rejecting it.

More importantly, however, society constantly interferes with mental patients' generation of "ideas." Indeed, if one regards behavior and emotions as proceeding from ideas, then getting people to change their ideas is the whole purpose of treatment. Involuntary commitment without any attempt to treat, despite the patients' pleas, violates their right to treatment. One might say that conventional therapies leave the patient's mental capacities intact. But before treatment he thinks one way; after successful treatment he thinks differently, and indeed we measure success by whether he is likely to return to his old habits. If this process generally does not raise First Amendment issues, even where treatment is compelled, I am dubious about placing purportedly consensual psychosurgery under First Amendment restraint.

In any event, the most that can be hoped for from First Amendment doctrine is a basis for insisting in court that serious procedures be scrutinized carefully. Viewing the psychosurgery problem from a broader policy perspective, we ought to accept the proposition that serious medical interventions should be closely scrutinized by someone regardless of whether it is grounded upon the Constitution. And, if the proposition is accepted, the case for a moratorium on the use of psychosurgery as an experimental therapy when patients cannot give full and free consent themselves is compelling. Not only do we lack good data on the efficacy of the procedures, we do not have any assurance that permitting the procedures in these settings will yield data. Nor can we be sure that such patients are not being asked to run risks for science by undergoing operations in which the risks exceed the likely gains.

When and if the situation is brought under better control, I do not see adequate reasons for barring psychosurgery entirely for such patients, either as an experimental therapy or, *a fortiori*, if it is a therapy whose efficacy has been fully established. There can be no question that the situation is rife with potential for abuse. For example, consider the situation of parents with a severely disturbed adolescent child who is ruining their lives both directly (he needs constant attention, beats up his siblings, the neighbors complain) and indirectly (through their guilt and their suffering because he suffers). Surely such parents are prone to therapy-shopping in the hope that somebody somewhere can do something. That they may consent to surgery with exceedingly low probability of success seems likely. Similarly, that the same haste may characterize the actions of those required to deal with highly disruptive mental patients cannot be gainsaid. But one cannot evaluate such situations without attention to the other hand. Supposing that highly qualified doctors from a variety of specialites ascertain that psychosurgery, albeit innovative, offers benefits worth risking in circumstances in which the therapeutic alternatives are futile and the prognosis one of endless suffering, I can see no reason for an absolute barrier to proceeding. We do not, for example, impose any barrier to such operations on defects of genetic or physical origins, where comparable potential for abuse exists.

It may also be desirable to impose procedural protections, such as requiring that no such operation on a person incapable of consent be done except upon court order. Lawyers in general have, and rightly so, a very high regard for process. Thinking about how to defend one's reasons for acting may halt many inappropriate actions in the embryo stage. Moreover, the focused attention of an organized proceeding may bring to light considerations which the proponents failed to consider. Surely the psychosurgery proposal at issue in the Michigan litigation shows that very questionable research projects can survive two levels of committee review. Besides, the protections provided by judicial process are likely to be effective where the decision called for is one the court must make infrequently. If 2,000 cases were presented yearly, judicial approval might become a rubber stamp. I think such a result improbable if two or three are weighed yearly.

155

If procedural protections are thought desirable a further regulatory question is whether judicial approval or some other mechanism should operate on a case-by-case basis, pursuant to standards so broad that they have no independent resolving power apart from precedents developed thereunder, or whether tighter standards should be maintained. The broad standards approach is frequently utilized in law in response to problems where linedrawing is difficult. For example, courts may refuse to enforce provisions of "unconscionable" contracts; what makes a contract unconscionable is left for particularized resolution in light of evolving case law.

I believe this regulatory solution is an unsatisfactory approach to psychosurgery. Unless some concrete standards are provided, the impulse to uphold medical judgments is too strong, particularly since the issue does not arise unless the patient's situation is such that performance of the procedure would be appropriate were the patient capable of assenting to it. To be sure, judicial or other oversight may add another layer of protection to assure compliance with that standard, a standard not now adequately enforced. But such oversight alone cannot come to grips with the principal public policy problem of protecting people who behave "differently" from being made more "normal," at some cost to their talents, because others think it best.

Judges have the same biases toward "normalcy" as the rest of us. The task is rather one of pledging ourselves to collective self-restraint in light of the history of social overresponse to, and misunderstanding of, people who are different. It is very hard to get adequate protection against overreaching unless some limitations on the procedures are divorced from an inquiry into whether the patient "really" would be better off as a consequence of their use. Or to put it differently, if enough protection is available without it, then formal legal procedures are probably uncalled for.

It is extremely difficult, however, to fashion easily applied rules that yield satisfactory results in the sense that they provide adequate protection against suppression of nonconformity in the name of "best interests," while at the same time not dooming people to lives of miserable discomfort to uphold principles drawn too broad. The problems in rule formulation are exacerbated because we know so little about the procedures and the effects they cause. For example, the question of whether and to what extent serious collateral consequences upon reasoning and affect are virtually inevitable in psychosurgery must surely weigh heavily in the balance. Consequently, my proposals for specific standards are proffered more as an invitation for criticism than with real confidence that they meet the needs of the situation in which people cannot, for any of the variety of the reasons discussed, give their full consent to psychosurgery.

First, the only considerations relevant to approving the use of such procedures if they carry high risks of irreversibly damaging the patient's general mental abilities are those that go to the patient's personal condition. That use of such procedures may facilitate accomplishment of the state's or a family's interest in preventing harmful behavior is not an independent justification for their use. Granted that we vaccinate people who object to it to protect others,[45] the difference in the degree of infringement involved makes such precedents different in kind.

As a practical matter, however, it may be hard in many instances to separate the two concerns for reasons discussed earlier. If a person is so violent that the state must put him under total restraint if the operation is not performed, is the harm to him from that confinement (as total isolation for any substantial period surely has negative impact on intellectual and emotional capacities) relevant in assaying his best interests? In general, medical intervention requires assessing alternatives. That the patient will die if nothing is done justifies risk taking. But in this case the alternatives asserted to make the risks acceptable are a function of social controls not the spread of disease. To allow their consideration permits the state interest in behavior control to be given indirect effect.

Second, no psychosurgical procedure causing substantial personality change or carrying serious risks should be done if the patient, regardless of how or why he may be incompetent to consent, indicates that he does not want the operation performed, particularly after reasonable efforts have been made (including full disclosure of risks) to explain the situation to him. This principle,

I believe, is the most durable protection possible against use of these procedures to crush people who are labeled "mad" because of a mixture of extreme social and political alienation from the community. Accepting this principle might go far to alleviate fears about political use of this technology. Whether it can be implemented, however, assumes the capacity to separate people who cannot consent into two groups: those who want or essentially have no opinion about the procedure, and those who do not want it done, even granting that their reasons for not wanting it may be irrational or produced by precisely the same aberrancy that is contemplated to be changed by the procedure. Even if this assumption is true, there are other practical problems. What of the patient who wants the procedure performed when he is calmed by tranquilizing drugs, but refuses it when he is his "normal" paranoid self? Similarly, what should be the response to the possibility of parental or spousal influence, when the patient says "yes" in their presence but hedges or expresses uncertainties when left alone?[46] Discussion of these issues could fill another chapter; for now let me simply record my view that they are manageable if not "solvable."

Underlying the principle is my belief that we have been too slow to consider the diversity of circumstances that may account for an individual's inability to proffer effective consent. Even within the category of committed mental patients, there are wide variations in individual conditions. There is simply no need to proscribe patients participation in decisions about their treatment. Moreover the doctrine of consent serves generally to authorize action. The reasons why we disable a person from saying yes need not also lead to a conclusion that he cannot say no. Unfortunately, focus on the "right to treatment" has obscured and may even undercut equally substantial problems of a right *not* to have treatment. The prevailing view, although there has been little litigation, is that "appropriate" treatment in mental institutions is for the doctors to decide once the propriety of supervision is established.

There are some signs of change in this approach. In *Winters* v. *Miller*[47] a court of appeals reversed summary judgment and remanded for trial the damage action of a Christian Scientist who was forced to take thorazine while in a mental hospital. Although the decision, is a limited one in many respects, the case is an important first step. Similarly, the revised New York Mental Hygiene Law, shows some legislative recognition of the need for separating issues of supervision from issues of treatment. The statute requires "consent" prior to surgery, electroconvulsive therapy, and innovative drug use.[48] Taking this pronouncement to reflect the state's public policy even prior to its effective date, a New York Supreme Court judge refused permission to administer shock treatments to a mentally ill person who refused them.[49]

This sliding scale approach to competency is not without difficulties, but it is basically sound. The law is used to vary the meaning of labels depending on the purpose for which the label is used. The hard practical problems with a sliding-scale approach to concern situations in which the state's fiscal purposes have to be given consideration. For example, if a patient expresses preference for life-long confinement at the state's expense rather than swallow a single pill or, more likely, insists that both choices are out of the question, we may well say, "Swallow and go home." Where the procedure to be used is drastic, involving not only attempted behavior alteration but also the possible loss of other mental capacities, we should draw the line at forced imposition despite the fact that from our perspective the patient and society would both be improved.

Third, and finally, we should not allow performance of serious innovative psychosurgical procedures on people who cannot themselves consent, whatever the therapeutic intent, unless there is clear evidence that organic brain damage is present. Such organic brain damage may be a prerequisite to demonstration that such procedures "work" within the framework of the medical model as I discussed it earlier. Even if that is not so, I still favor the limitation where the patient cannot himself consent and the procedure is not fully tested. Such a rule may seem harsh in some instances, but it does protect against overweighting environmental factors in deciding that psychosurgery is appropriate. Granted that organic pathology may ultimately be turned into a fiction by more sensitive brain-monitoring devices, nonetheless it is for now a useful fiction.

As to operations which have been tested adequately, I think that familial or guardian consent, coupled with patient nonrefusal after full disclosure of risks, should suffice for whatever court approval, if such procedures are deemed necessary. Allowing operations even in these circumstances opens up avenues of possible abuse. Nonetheless, to say that public policy commands that we leave people to their fates, regardless of what that fate may be, supports the wrong principle. That abuse is so hard to check underlines strongly the central importance of effective regulation both of whether the operation works and whether its administration is appropriate in the particular instance, apart from issues of consent.

Psychosurgery and Penal Policy

Public discussion of psychosurgery has focused heavily on the appropriateness of using such techniques to rehabilitate violent criminal offenders. Perhaps the reason for the focus, along with our mixture of fascination and anxiety about crime, was the assertion of Drs. Mark and Ervin that many participants in the Detroit riots in 1967 suffered from brain conditions that would profit from such treatment, an assertion long since recanted. In any event, so far as I know, very few psychosurgical procedures have been done on prisoners in the United States.[50] Moreover, insofar as psychosurgery has been used on violent persons, it has typically been done where the patient was epileptic. Despite understandable fears about misuse of medicine in the prisons, it seems mental patients run greater risks of exposure to this technology, just as was the case in prefrontal lobotomy days.

I believe it very unlikely that we shall ever make much use of psychosurgery as a rehabilitative technique because it is so unspecific in its effects. But the issues, although academic, are interesting. I think it clear that we should not now allow any such procedure to be done without an inmate's consent. Without much better evidence concerning the efficacy of the procedures, to impose them would be to convert criminal conviction into a license for medical experimentation on a victim, not a patient. Granted that a good deal of rehabilitative experimentation is tolerated though intrusive, such as mandatory group therapy, differences in degree at some point become differences in kind. Psychosurgery crosses that line because of irresistibility, irreversibility, and prospects of serious collateral damage. Strong arguments could be made that any such mandatory treatment was unconstitutional on a variety of grounds, of which cruel and unusual punishment is probably the strongest.[51]

Second, I think it also reasonably clear that any imposed use of such procedures should be rejected even if they are ascertained to be effective—in the sense that they work at levels of risk doctors and nonincarcerated patients deem it appropriate to accept—so long as there is any substantial risk of failure or of collateral effects. A goal of preventing recurrence of criminal behavior does not justify the use of means which blunt and destroy the person's other capacities. To be sure, prison may often lead to this same result, but that argues more for penal reform than substitution of comparable evils on the grounds that they are cheaper. Moreover, although prison may work such destruction and change, it often does not do so. As a practical matter, I doubt that there is much prospect of forced use of these procedures on offenders even if they are deemed effective. It is more likely that persons who are treatable will be thought not responsible for their behavior and remitted to the mental health process. The standards I have discussed earlier would protect their refusal to consent in that setting.

Current practical questions relating to psychosurgery in the prisons do not concern mandatory treatment, but rather whether special standards are required to limit the circumstances in which inmates or potential inmates may consent to therapy. I believe the case for such standards is compelling. As with institutionalized mental patients, there are strong reasons for fearing overreaching. The situation is slightly different in that the inmate is presumptively competent to assess his own situation. Nonetheless, the decision to be treated may not reflect desire to have it but simply a distaste for alternatives perceived to be equally unfair, i.e. prison.

Although I do not believe that hard choices are coerced ones, there is a special danger in giving an "easy" way out since it removes the social pressure for constant reevaluation of why the alternatives are structured as they are. In the case of penal policy, there can be no forgetting that despite the attention paid to crime, and indeed because of it, sensitive estimations of the minimum levels of force necessary to accomplish our purposes are rarely acted upon. If public policy permits, or worse, encourages wide-scale use of cheap but destructive control mechanisms, the underlying questions of why we put people to such choices will receive less attention.

Other objections to the use of inmates as experimental subjects flow from the demands of public safety. Psychosurgical procedures must be better evaluated, and yet adequate assessment of their efficacy is not feasible if a person is kept under lock and key. On the current evidence, the public is inadequately protected if violent offenders are simply operated upon and released. We have some basis for thinking that the calming effects of psychosurgical procedures are not long lasting, as Vaughan notes in Chapter 2.

Thus I believe that proffering such procedures to inmates or potential inmates is wrong. The latter practice may be thought somewhat less coercive, in that the patient consents before he is institutionalized and suffers whatever dependency results from that process, but it is equally inappropriate. Unfortunately, even the newer penal codes allow this practice, because they usually authorize imposing as a condition of probation that the offender seek specific medical treatment, without qualification as to whether the mode of treatment is generally recognized as effective.[52] Although I know of no data indicating how frequently such referrals occur, newspapers occasionally report that some judge has agreed to let a prisoner go free only if he turns himself over to a doctor.

If psychosurgical procedures are ascertained to be effective remedies for violent outbursts, in the sense that doctors on adequate evidence find the benefits outweigh the risks even for patients under no threat of restraint, and the procedures are a recognized therapy for such patients, then the issues are much more complex. On the one hand, the fact that procedures work cannot vitiate concern for the quality of consent within prison walls. Some people are terribly frightened by their violent proclivities; others clearly do not care at all, and for them therapy is simply a means of escape. On the other hand, granting the possibilities for abuse, I think it unfair to disable people from consenting to procedures that are "efficacious" even if they were not facing criminal sanctions. To do so adds loss of rights to medical treatment to the general consequences of penal conviction.

A possible response to this problem is to say that performance of the procedure will be given no dispositional significance whatever. I do not believe, however, that such stringency is warranted. If a person's criminal behavior was substantially related to a mental condition (albeit nonexculpating), and that condition has been altered so that he is no longer dangerous, it would be inhumane to insist on further incarceration simply to prove the point. Unlike prisoner participation in nontherapeutic experimentation, where we can insist that volunteering may make no or little difference, performance of the procedure goes right to the heart of why we insist upon restraints.

Consequently, my tentative thinking is that the following lines should be drawn. First, as to tested procedures performed with some frequency on consenting patients not immediately facing penal sanctions, consent by inmates should be allowed. Second, consent to innovative operations should be allowed only where there is clear evidence of organic brain damage and, as a practical matter, the nature of the operation is such that establishing the benefits and the risks of the procedure on persons not facing penal or comparable restraint is impossible.

Finally, I wish to close by discussing briefly a problem I do not believe we shall face, at least not in the near future. Suppose psychosurgery, or more probably other physical brain therapies like ESB, are developed with such precision that the procedure interferes only with the actor's capacity to behave criminally, and does not otherwise affect him. Frankly I doubt the premise, given the subtleties of what conduct is called criminal for society. Criminal violence involves wrongful aggressiveness, larceny is wrongful acquisitiveness, rape can be wrongful seduction. We do not find these behaviors in their basic form offensive; quite the contrary, they are vital parts of our community. Only their extreme manifestations are called criminal, and I think it unlikely that behavioral therapies can trace the shifting line of what society at any point in time finds extreme. Nonetheless, I shall consider the issue briefly because it figures so large in public debates on the propriety of developing these techniques.

Arguments can be made against forced imposition of even such precise instruments of rehabilitation. First, there is the problem of the "dangerous precedent." Concepts like "capacity" are inherently ambiguous; one can nearly always claim some marginal alteration of human potention. Under the pressure of mounting expenses for programs that do not work, the impulse is strong to characterize increasingly severe collateral damage as marginal, in order to allow programs that do work.

Second, many might claim an absolute preference for working *through* the person, rather than *on* him, in an effort to maintain lines between coerced persuasion and coercion simpliciter. Drawing such a line reflects the utility of deviance. Historically, expansion of personal freedom from constraints in behaving as one chooses has often depended upon the fact that there are enough people who want to behave in similar fashion and no practical ways of stopping them. Recognition of the futility of sanctions sparks the reappraisal that they are inappropriate. A current example of this process at work is the slow passage of marijuana use from serious crime, to criminal-medical problem, and probably ultimately to a matter of personal choice. To allow quick and effective means of keeping people from doing what you do not want them to do undercuts this vital method for forcing recognition that community morality has changed to the extent that social response to the behavior must also change.

Both considerations are important, but I think it wrong to overstate them. Certainly it is absurd to think that the community is likely to regard outbursts of undirected rage resulting in mass murder, or sexual desires so uncontrolled that they result in a series of rapes, as within the range of "normal" behavior. If it were possible to excise the particular behavior without having any other effects, I cannot see any absolute moral barrier to doing so. The problems are those of degree—how serious the behavior, how intensive the therapy, and so on. However, we will not be forced to make such choices in the near future, and it may be that we will never hone so finely the consequences of therapeutic intervention.

164

NOTES

1. Problems of behavior control, particularly legal restraints upon its compulsory imposition, have become topics of major concern for legal writers. See, e.g., James Gobert, "Psychosurgery, Conditioning, and the Prisoner's Right to Refuse Rehabilitation," *University of Virginia Law Review* 61 (1975): 155-196; Michael Shapiro, "Legislating the Control of Behavior Control: Autonomy and the Coercive Use of Organic Therapies," *Southern California Law Review* 47 (1974): 237-356; Ralph Schwitzgebel, "Limitations on the Coercive Treatment of Offenders," *Criminal Law Bulletin* 8 (1972): 267-320; David Wexler, "Therapeutic Justice," *Minnesota Law Review* 57 (1972) 289-338; David Wexler, "Token and Taboo; Behavior Modification, Token Economics, and the Law," *California Law Review* 61 (1973): 81-109; Student Note, " 'Conditioning and Other Techniques Used to Treat? 'Rehabilitate?' 'Demolish?' Prisoners and Mental Patients," *Southern California Law Review* 45 (1972): 616-681; Symposium, "Psychosurgery," *Boston University Law Review* 54 (1974): 215-354.

The leading federal cases discussing behavior control are *Clonce* v. *Richardson*, 379 F. Supp. 338 (W. D. Mo. 1974); *Knecht* v. *Gillman*, 448 F.2d 1136 (8th Cir. 1973); *Mackey* v. *Procunier* 477 F.2d 877 (9th Cir. 1973); *United States* v. *Alexander* 471 F.2d 1923 (D.C. Cir. 1972) (dictum) (Bazelon J.).

2. See, e.g., Ore. Revised Stat. § 677.190 (23) (1953); Ore. Revised Stat. § § 426.700-755 (1974 Chapters Replaced); Cal. Welfare & Institutions Code § § 5325 (g); 5326.3 (1975 Supp.); Cal Penal Code § § 2670-2680 (1975) Supp.).

The Oregon statutes require committee screening before any psychosurgery is performed. The California legislation applies only to institutionalized persons.

3. National Research Act of 1974, § 202 (c), 88 Stat 342. It requires the newly established National Commission for the Protection of Human Subjects of Biomedical and Behavioral Research to study the use of psychosurgery in the United States for the five-year period ending 1972.

4. Hearings on S. 974, S. 878, and S.J. Res. 71 before the Subcomm. on Health of the Sen. Comm. on Labor and Public Welfare, 93d Cong. 1st Sess. (1973).

5. *Kaimowiz* v. *Department of Mental Health*, Civ. No. 73-19434AW (Cir. Ct., Wayne City, Mich., 1973).

6. Ore. Revised Stats. § 426.700(6), (1974 Chapters Replaced).

7. Dr. Peter Breggin, whose protests concerning psychosurgery have fired much of the controversy, gave this definition as paraphrased by the Court, in his Kaimowitz testimony, slip opinion at 10.

8. Cal. Welfare & Institutions Code § 5325 (g), (1975 Supp.).

9. Robert Michels, "Ethical Issues of Psychological and Psychotherapeutic Means of Behavior Control," *Hastings Center Report* 3, no. 2 (1973): 11-13.

10. The three definitions differ in several respects. For example, is behavior control by electric stimulation of the brain (ESB) "Psychosurgery"? Dr. Breggin's definition of psychosurgery would seemingly comprehend ESB, since tissue is destroyed to "control emotions or behavior." The Oregon formulation probably excludes ESB because the destruction of tissue is not "designed," but is rather an inevitable consequence of implantation. Note, however, that Oregon's definition includes the destruction of abnormal brain tissue causing aberrant behavior. Dr. Breggin's does not.

In discussing this problem with doctors, my experience is that they do not regard the problem of definition as substantial. However, when pressed on whether they characterize as psychosurgery operations for pain generally, pain in phantom limbs, or for behavior clearly attributable to epilepsy, it becomes clear that differences in usage exist among them.

11. Even noninnovative surgery can be very dangerous. See Charles Child, "Surgical Intervention." *Scientific American* 229, no. 3(1973): 90-98, for a table (p. 97) showing

a range of .3 deaths per 10,000 operations (tonsilectomy without adenoidectomy) to 1,328.2 deaths per 10,000 operations (exploratory laparotomy or celiotomy) among the most commonly done procedures in 1969.

12. Judith Swazey and Rene Fox, "The Clinical Moratorium," in *Experimentation with Human Subjects*, edited by Paul Freund. New York: Braziller, 1970, pp. 315-323. Nine of the first twelve patients died during the operation or within a week thereafter. The procedures were done between 1912 and 1928. Learning from experience, surgeons now do the operation with far greater success.

13. Between December 3, 1967, and May 11, 1969, 132 heart-transplant operations were done throughout the world. Eighty-one patients died within two months; another fourteen died within six months. See *Cardiac Replacement*, A Report by the Ad Hoc Task Force on Cardiac Replacement, National Heart Institute. Washington, D.C.: U.S. Government Printing Office, 1969.

14. Peter Breggin, "The Return of Lobotomy," *Congressional Record*, 118th Cong., E 1603, E 1605, Feb. 24, 1972.

15. Vernon Mark and Frank Ervin, *Violence and the Brain*. New York: Harper & Row, 1970.

16. Dr. Rodin believed the book was at fault, and that he had been "misled by the literature." Memo Rodin to Gottlieb, August 9, 1972.

17. "Ethical Guidelines for Clinical Investigation." *Opinions and Reports of the Judicial Council*. Chicago: American Medical Association, 1969, pp. 9-11.

18. Irving Cooper, *The Victim is Always the Same*. New York: Harper & Row, 1970.

19. The only justification for so doing is if one treats protection of the doctor-patient relation as the sole interest at stake. Where the physician perceives himself to be experimenting, that relation is inevitably threatened even where performance of the procedure is justified solely by therapeutic considerations. Therefore, to justify running those risks, the physician must design the experiment competently.

20. As Dr. Vaughan notes in Chapter 2, differences in diagnostic criteria for schizophrenia make comparisons between English and American experience with psychosurgery difficult.

21. See, generally, Fred Inbau and Jon Waltz, *Medical Jurisprudence*. New York: Macmillan, 1971.

22. See, e.g., *Fiorentino* v. *Wenger*, 26 App. Div. 2d 693, 272 N.Y.S. 2d 557 (2d Dept. 1966), reversed as to def. hosp. 19 N.Y. 2d 407, 280 N.Y.S. 2d 373, 227 N.E. 2d 296 (1967); see also *Leech* v. *Bralliar*, 275 F. Supp. 897 (D. Ariz. 1967).

23. See e.g., *Ardoline* v. *Keegan*, 140 Conn. 552, 102 A. 2d 352 (1954).

24. See, generally, Jon Waltz and Thomas Scheuneman, "Informed Consent to Therapy," *Northwestern University Law Review* 64 (1970): 628-650; Comment, "Informed Consent in Medical Malpractice," *California Law Review* 55 (1967): 1396-1418.

See also *Canterbury* v. *Spence*, 464 F. 2d 772 (D.C. Cir. 1972)(nondisclosure of percent risk of paralysis requires jury trial). Whether the duty to disclose has been breached is usually analyzed as a question of negligence. The difficult problems, occasioning a flood of legal commentary, are whether standards of disclosure should be set by reference to practices of other doctors, doctors in the locality, and so on, or what a "reasonable" man would disclose.

25. See *Board of Medical Registration and Examination* v. *Kaadt*, 76 N.E. 2d. 669 (Ind. 1948) as an example of its use. See also Jay Katz with Alexander Capron and Eleanor Glass, eds., *Experimentation with Human Beings*. New York: Russell Sage Foundation, 1972, pp. 9-66, for interesting materials on the "Jewish Chronic Disease Hospital Case" in which physicians were disciplined for injecting live cancer cells into chronically ill patients without their knowledge or consent.

26. See *National Research Act of 1974*, 212, 88 Stat 342, establishing an "Ethics

Guidance Program," and mandating that federal grantees establish institutional review boards.

27. See *Fiorentino* v. *Wenger*, 19 N.Y. 2d 407, 280 N.Y.S. 2d 373, 227 N.E. 2d 296 (1967).

28. Cf. *Tunk* v. *Regents of University of California*, 60 Cal. 2d 92, 383 P. 2d 441, 32 Cal. Rptr. 33 (1966).

29. See 21 U.S.C. § § 321; 352; 355 (a), (b), (e), (i), (j). For an excellent overview of drug regulation see Richard Merrill, "Compensation for Prescription Drug Injuries," *University of Virginia Law Review* 59 (1973): 1-28.

30. The best known is Richardson-Merrell's marketing of MER/29 despite evidence which it failed to report that the drug caused serious side effects in animal studies. See *Toole* v. *Richardson-Merrell Inc.*, 251 Cal. App. 689, Cal. Reptr. 398 (1st. Dist. 1967).

31. See Merrill "Compensation," n. 29.

32. 154 Cal. App. 2d 560, 317 P. 2d 170, 179-180 (1st Dist. 1957). Recent malpractice decisions may impose new restraints on physicians' deviations from manufacturers' recommendations as to drug use. See, e.g., *Mulder* v. *Parke-Davis & Co.*, 288 Minn. 332, 181 Nw. 2d 882 (1970). The key issue is whether the physician may justify departing from the FDA-approved instructions simply by reference to the practice of other physicians in the area, and, if not, what other evidence is necessary.

33. In this connection, there are useful analogies to be found in the FDA's treatment of medical "devices." Unlike drugs, devices may be marketed without costly prescreening to assure their safety and efficacy. The statutory definition of a device, however, overlaps closely that of the term "drug." *Compare* 21 U.S.C. § 321 (g) *with* 21 USC § 321 (h). Drugs are "articles" intended for use in the diagnosis, cure, mitigation, treatment, or prevention of disease in man or other animals, or intended to affect the structure or any function of the body of man or other animals. Devices are "instruments, apparatus, and contrivances" intended for either of those same two purposes.

In *United States* v. *Bacto-Unidisk*, 394 U.S. 784 (1969), the Supreme Court construed the term "drug" very broadly. A diagnostic aid impregnated with antibiotics was held to be a "drug," not a "device," and thus subject to FDA rules requiring prescreening. The language of the Court's opinion is broad enough, moreover, to permit characterizing an electrode used in electric brain stimulation or phsychosurgery as a drug, a course which, if taken, would require manufacturers to develop clinical evidence of the safety of the procedures for which it is intended.

The FDA has made *little* use of its expanded power, however, despite its recognition that unsafe medical instruments are a serious problem. The reason is that the "device" industry is so fragmented, and the prospects of profits so low, given the small quantities needed, that manufacturers in many instances would stop production rather than bear the huge costs that compliance with the "new drug" rules entails. The practical problem is to get anyone to manufacture devices.

34. Ore. Revised Stats. § § 426.700-755 (1974 Chapters Replaced).

35. See Cooper, *The Victim is Always the Same*, n. 18, for a moving report on the psychological consequences for patient and family of repeated exposure to conventional therapies which do not work.

36. See David Wexler, Stanley Scoville, et al., "The Administration of Psychiatric Justice: Theory and Practice in Arizona," *Arizona Law Reivew* 13 (1971): 1, 66-69, 189-200, for chilling accounts of common practices.

37. Cosmetic plastic surgery is perhaps the best example of the use of serious surgical procedures where nothing is organically wrong with the patient. Moreover, in some circumstances such surgery may be used only because the patient's environment cannot be changed. For example, suppose a child has a physical abnormality which is organically harmless, but makes him an object of harmful ridicule by his peer group. One cannot practically change the others. Should the child have an operation?

38. American Law Institute, *Model Penal Code* § 4.01(2) (Proposed Off. Draft, 1962). The principle serves to defeat claims of criminal irresponsibility (insanity).

39. Although attempting suicide is not a crime in most states, the likelihood that one may commit suicide is commonly utilized as a basis for involuntary committment. See, e.g., N.Y. Mental Hygiene Law §§ 31.39, 31.41, 31.43. Moreover, assisting a person to kill himself is generally some form of criminal homicide, either by special statute, e.g., N.Y. Penal Law §§ 125.25(1)(b), or by application of general homicide provisions, e.g., *People* v. *Roberts*, 211 Mich. 187, 178 N.W. 690 (1920).

40. See Joanne Stern, "Medical Treatment and the Teenager: The Need for Parental Consent," *Clearinghouse Review* 7 (May 1973): 1. 1-5. State legislation authorizing doctors to provide medical care to minors without parental consent is common as to venereal disease and contraception. See Harriet Pilpel and Nancy Wechsler, "Birth Control, Teenagers, and the Law," *Family Planning Perspectives* 1 (Spring 1969): 29.

41. *Physical Manipulation of the Brain at 18*, Hastings Center Report, Special Supplement, May 1973, p. 18.

42. *Kaimowitz* v. *Department of Mental Health*, Civ. No. 73-19434AW (Cir. Ct., Wayne City, Mich., 1973) m. 5.

43. Ibid., Slip opinion at 40.

44. Ibid., Slip opinion at 36.

45. *Jacobsen* v. *Massachusetts*, 197 U.S. 11 (1905).

46. For a difficult problem of this sort, see *Physical Manipulation of the Brain*, m. 4, p. 14.

47. 446 F.2d 65 (2d Cir.) cert. denied 404 U.S. 985 (1971).

48. N.Y. Mental Hygiene Law § 15.03(4). The statute leaves open whether the patient must himself consent, or whether consent may be obtained by proxy.

49. *New York City Health & Hospitals Corp.* v. *Stein*, 70 Misc. 2d 944, 355 N.U.S. 2d. 461 (Sup. Ct., N.Y. City, 1972). The court found that the patient "had the mental capacity to know and understand whether she wishes to consent to electroshock therapy."

50. Operations were apparently performed on three California prisoners in 1965. See "State Tries Brain Surgery to Control Violent Prisoners," *Sacramento Bee*, February 27, 1972, pp. 1, 16. The results were described as mixed. One patient showed marked improvement, another fair results, and the third little or no change. The patient with "marked improvement" was paroled and then convicted of robbery in Montana in 1969.

51. In *Mackey* v. *Propcunier*, 477 F.2d 877 (9th Cir. 1973), plaintiff, a prisoner, alleged that state prison officials had administered succinychlorine to him without his consent as part of a program of experimentation. The drug causes temporary total paralysis, and, as used, makes the patient exceedingly frightened because he cannot breathe. The Court held it a potentially actionable violation of his rights.

52. See, e.g., N.Y. Penal Law § 65.10.

JOEL S. MEISTER, Ph. D.

6 / The Need for Policy

THE PSYCHOSURGERY CONFLICT has become a classic example of the politicization of medicine. Nor is it an isolated example, for the social role of medicine is changing rapidly. The medical profession is becoming more secularized and the society is becoming more medicalized. Thus psychosurgery is at once both a medical technique and a sociological concept. It describes a surgical procedure and yet is no different from other procedures which are called, simply, neurosurgery. It is a treatment meant to change behaviors rather than to remove diseased portions of the body; yet, similar procedures also meant to change behavior—say, to relieve the tremors of Parkinsonism—are not described as psychosurgery. The term "psychosurgery" clearly has been reserved only for certain behaviors, namely, those labeled deviant or abnormal. The pattern of normality over against which behavioral deviance is perceived consists of the web of laws, norms, customs, and habits by which social life is ordered. My remarks in this chapter are predicated on the assumption that psychosurgery is inherently a political act in the broad sense in which politics refers to the definition of the social good as well as to the resolution of conflicts over control of the social goods. Others have called psychosurgery a political act in the narrowest sense—a technique for controlling political opposition. This latter meaning may be argued on its merits but is not an assumption made here.

The politicization of medicine goes well beyond psychosurgery. The economic base of medical care is not the paying private patient but the third-party institution and the federal subsidy. Medical care has simply become too expensive for even middle-class patients. The socialization of the cost of care as well as of research and training has brought medicine fully into the public domain. Against the claims to professional autonomy made by medical organizations there is developing a consensus that health, and consequently, medical care are rights as fundamental as those to life and liberty and are not to be limited by one's ability to pay. And so the trend in medicine generally is toward greater public accountability and more external control.

The fruits of research include promising treatments and palliatives for an impressive array of mental ills. Major tranquilizers have made possible the deinstitutionalization of thousands of mental hospital patients, and amphetamine drugs have been extensively used to treat children with minimal brain dysfunction (MBD). In the latter case, it appears that the illness category of MBD emerged as a response to the development of a medical treatment for a variety of behavioral disturbances once known as hyperactivity. In other words, the development of a specifically organic treatment evoked an ostensibly organically based disorder. This is what I call the medicalization of deviance, whereby genetic or other organic causes come to replace psychosocial variables in the explanation of deviance from normative behavior, in part as a consequence of the development of organic means of controlling behavior, and not because we have actually discovered a piece of the body that doesn't work right.

But medicine is also becoming politicized because it is indeed discovering more about how our brains function and more about how to manipulate those functions. Psychosurgery results from the increasing technical sophistication and more inclusive body of knowledge of medicine, and this growing presence of medical technology must be added to the catalog of political issues raised by psychosurgery. Given the recognition of a public role in the development and assessment of new technologies and new uses for existing technologies, it remains for us to devise effective means for the social control of medical innovation which will not stifle the innovators or the very process of innovation.

Psychosurgery has been touted as the "surgery of violence." Considering that as a treatment for the assaultive individual, psychosurgery was devised and promoted during one of the most violent periods in our recent history, it is worth making a brief review of the legacy of this recent past. On the far side of the 1960s, we find ourselves now in a period of reaction to the discontent and turmoil of those years. We seem to be trying to "forget" as quickly as possible the urban racial rebellion, the moral and military catastrophe of Vietnam, the student revolt, the efflorescence of a counterculture, the assassinations, and the public violence and spectacle attending all these events. The "Great Society" rhetoric of change and progress has gone flat, and some of the social programs themselves have been dismantled.

The memories, and especially the fears, linger; the fear of uncontrollable mobs, children, and governments. Influential members of our intellectual and academic communities are dismayed by the apparent ineffectiveness of the very programs they once supported. It is likely, they suggest, that a political, governmental response to social problems, in the New Deal tradition, is inappropriate; that our discontents lie beyond the reach of such programs, however grand their scope. A more convincing "cure" may be just what the doctor orders. An eminent neurosurgeon first made the connection between psychosurgery and social violence, not a fearful or ignorant public. Despite subsequent qualification and reconsideration, the public remains confused—and rightly so— about the potential uses, the motives for use, and the effects of this technology. Psychosurgery has become a volatile issue because it is inextricably bound to this social context. Following the apparent failure to manipulate well our social environment, we are all the more willing to focus our concerns and our talents on the internal environments of individuals, an orientation which seems congenial to social order.

Had we only to consider the scientific merits of the procedures and the ethics of human experimentation, the problem would still be formidable. We need to address the questions of how the limits

171

of our knowledge about brain processes should affect psycho-surgical practices; of the criteria and process by which an innova-tive technique becomes accepted therapy; of the conditions under which the therapy is indicated; of the protection of patients through informed consent, and so on. We must consider the implications of the dilemma caused by our desire to protect patients and our desire to encourage research and effective therapy. My point is that we must do this and more, because all the broad issues affect our answers to the seemingly more specific ones, and all of them are legitimate. In this chapter I shall examine several areas of concern that bear directly on the regulation of psychosurgery. These include the definition of psychosurgery, its potential social abuse, its experimental status, and the specific groups to whom *policy* might be addressed.

Defining Psychosurgery

Psychosurgery must be specifically defined in order to clarify to what procedures regulations would apply. To make policy, we must know as precisely as possible the procedures and conditions of treatment that are in question. I shall discuss four approaches to defining psychosurgery. The first two are based on the *motives* for treatment, the third on the *conditions* warranting treatment, and the fourth on the *effects* of treatment. While each approach involves some ambiguity, I shall argue in favor of concentrating on the effects of psychosurgery.

Let us first consider psychosurgery as "psychiatric neurosur-gery," or as neurosurgery used to treat psychiatric illness, or more generally as "the neurosurgical treatment of behavioral dis-orders."[3] By this definition, the same procedure used to treat epileptic seizures or Parkinsonism would not be considered an instance of psychosurgery.

There are three principal objections to this approach. It is very difficult to know when a procedure is used for psychiatric purposes, and the domain of psychiatric illnesses is not well defined. One psychiatrist's diagnosis of "mental illness" may be another's "rational response to a sick environment."[8] We are not in a position to settle classifications of psychiatric conditions, nor can we wait until the psychiatric profession reaches a publicly acknowledged consensus on a range of respectable opinions. A definition of psychosurgery ought not be at the mercy of these theoretical debates. More practically, there are some kinds of psychiatric neurosurgery, including those meant to reduce or eliminate pain, that do not seem controversial in the same way or for the same reason that other kinds do.

If defining the appropriate purpose is difficult, discerning the motive in the surgeon's mind is even harder. The surgeon may have mixed motives, such as operating to control epileptic seizures and at the same time intending to eliminate attacks of uncontrollable rage, perhaps with the same lesion. If the surgeon has a psychiatric motive but wishes to avoid strict protocols for psychosurgery, he can claim another motive. In precisely those cases that are controversial, it would be difficult to specify a given operation as an instance of psychosurgery.

Another objection arises from the recognition that there may well be procedures that are not psychiatric in purpose but which entail similar liabilities. Many neurosurgical procedures carry the potential liabilities of memory loss, diminished affect, and reduced creativity on which much attention in the psychosurgery controversy centers.[7] Yet these neurosurgical procedures are not equated with psychosurgery. While these other purposes—curtailing pain, or seizures, or Parkinsonism—seem to justify the attendant loss of mental functions, perhaps the risk-benefit question should be asked explicitly by means of protocols appropriate for psychiatric neurosurgery. Furthermore, if the real motive of the surgeon or family or hospital is psychosurgical—perhaps to produce docility in an obstreperous patient—and if the patient also happens to have epilepsy with seizures, then the jeopardy of corrupt treatment and evaluation is all the greater if some neurosurgical procedures are free of psychosurgical regulation whenever allegedly used for nonpsychiatric motives. Finally, there are serious difficulties in writing any guidelines, regulations, or laws that define psychosurgery according to the motive for which a procedure is used. We should much prefer that any professional, administrative, or judicial body assess a practice according to criteria based on acts, not intentions. Certainly the grounds of judgment would be more easily accessible to public inspection.

A variation of the definition by motive is to restrict the range of psychiatric illnesses to those with organic brain pathology.[6] The advantage here is that in principle the brain pathology can be verified objectively, and thus the question of motive altered. Instead of asking what the surgeon's motive is, the question becomes what his motive ought to be, or is justified in being, given the pathology. The effect would be to tie psychosurgery more closely to the biological branches of clinical medicine. This strategy has its own serious difficulties. Defining an anatomical or functional characteristic of the brain as pathological is almost as difficult as defining mental illness, and is just as open to controversy. Herbert Vaughan has reviewed this issue at length in Chapter 2. Perhaps brain abnormality can be defined according to statistical distributions, but to call an abnormality bad, and thus pathological, is a further step, and one difficult to justify in some cases. And no two brains are alike. If a brain structure or function is found to be associated with some behavior disliked by certain people, that brain characteristic could be declared pathological and the person considered a candidate for psychosurgery without warrant.

This approach, like the first one, would also fail to regulate many other practices of psychiatric neurosurgery that are not restricted to treating psychiatric conditions involving brain pathology. Regulations might state that psychiatric neurosurgery in all cases other than those with brain pathology ought to be proscribed. But then we are reduced to our original definition and can only distinguish between legitimate and illegitimate psychosurgery. Although our aim is to make such distinctions, the definition remains inadequate.

Psychosurgery could be defined instead by a specified list of psychiatric conditions with indicated neurosurgical treatments. For example, "psychosurgery is the neurosurgical treatment of depression, obsessive-compulsive neurosis, and unmotivated, involuntary aggression." Surgery for pain and seizures would be excluded on the grounds that they do not need regulation by psychosurgical guidelines. This is one way out of the theoretical controversies over definition of psychiatric illnesses. It avoids the problem of determining motives. It has the advantage of regulating specific procedures when the professional community and the public believe there is good reason for singling them out as problematic. This approach based on conditions warranting treatment has two serious flaws. First, this definition of psychosurgery would not apply to, and therefore would not regulate, any psychiatric uses of neurosurgery not on the list. Thus it would have to stipulate that "all other psychosurgical practices are illegitimate," and again we would be stuck with an inadequate definition. Second, this approach requires the development of a consensus of the professional community regarding procedures needing regulation. Yet one of the main purposes of guidelines is to warn in advance of procedures likely to be dangerous.

The most promising, most comprehensive approach is based on the effects of psychosurgery. While the danger here is that this definition could be too inclusive, it would allow us to discriminate among specific procedures. Psychosurgery would be defined by a listing of neurosurgical procedures that have direct effects on thought, emotion, or behavior. Any new procedure with such effects would automatically be added to the list. Guidelines for each procedure would then distinguish between their use for noncontroversial and for controversial purposes, prescribing protocols, indications, and so on. Psychosurgery would cease to be a special domain, and attention would focus on procedures that might have direct psychological effects, whatever their purpose. Each procedure would be dealt with on the merits of its therapeutic effectiveness and attendant dangers.

This approach has several advantages. First, threats to personal integrity latent in some neurological procedures would be taken into account by regulations even when those procedures are used for purposes other than psychiatric ones. Second, the motive of the surgeon would be irrelevant to the indication or proscription of the procedure. Third, the medical status of the procedures in various contexts could be codified and stated explicitly in the interest of legal clarity. Fourth, attention would be called to the empirical issues in each case, not to ideological ones. The question would not be whether psychosurgery is good or bad, but whether these procedures are worthwhile and safeguarded in a specific context.

All brain surgery has direct psychological effects. Regulations based on this definition would extend beyond our current, essentially political, conception of psychosurgery. But by emphasizing a primary concern with psychological effects and by calling attention to areas of controversy, this definition should allow us to make appropriate distinctions within the entire domain of procedures having "direct effects on thought, emotion, or behavior." In doing away with "psychosurgery" as a useful category we would bring about the return of a well-oriented empirical study, concentrating on the problems of employing and evaluating an experimental therapy. There is a loss to be sustained, however, in abandoning the term "psychosurgery." It has been more popular with the public than with the medical community, and it connotes the public's perception of psychosurgery as a form of behavior control for nontherapeutic purposes. The danger is that regulations may omit important, nontherapeutic issues from their purview.

The Experimental Status of Psychosurgery

The sense in which psychosurgery is experimental is itself a matter of debate. "Experimental" is often contrasted with "therapeutic" to describe a procedure used primarily to gain knowledge, without reasonable expectation of an immediate therapeutic benefit. Psychosurgery is not experimental in this sense because every reported case involves specific therapeutic intentions. It is more accurate to consider whether it is an experimental therapy; whether it poses the kinds of questions that indicate the need for experimental clinical controls and monitoring.

Those who claim that psychosurgery is not experimental point out that all the surgical techniques involved, including the stereotaxic placement of electrodes, are standard operating procedures for other treatment purposes. There is nothing experimental about putting a lesion in the desired area, although there are constant technical improvements in the accuracy of these techniques. Nor is psychosurgery a life-threatening procedure; from this point of view it is comparatively very safe. Nor is it true that we lack follow-up studies. Such studies exist,[1,10] and while their sufficiency and accuracy may be arguable, they do provide some longitudinal evidence of relief of specific symptoms, lack of deleterious side effects, and good postoperative social adjustment.[1,3,4] They also provide some indications of the range of conditions responsive to psychosurgical treatment. Schizophrenics, for example, do not seem to respond to psychosurgery. Although these studies indicate some promising results, when we consider that there are no generally accepted standards of psychiatric evaluation and presently no mechanisms for systematic evaluation of psychosurgical practices, the available clinical evidence seems inadequate to warrant general acceptance of psychosurgery as a standard therapy.

The use of these techniques to treat a range of psychiatric illnesses is indeed experimental in several ways. We do not know how and why psychosurgery works because our knowledge of the brain is limited. We do not know how aspirin works, either, but in the case of psychosurgery effectiveness is difficult to predict, the range of possible side effects is very wide, and they do not "wear off." The unpredictability of effects is partly due to difficulty in placing lesions accurately, but more significantly it results from the still-mysterious complexity of brain functions and the often-bewildering relations between brain structure and environment. While more studies will be helpful in answering these questions, another consequence of the experimental nature of psychosurgery is that there remain theoretical difficulties in defining controlled longitudinal studies for mentally ill persons that would identify subtle side effects associated with the surgery. Finally, we do not yet have acceptable criteria for evaluating patients in diagnosis and follow-up. Our categories of mental illness are not sufficiently defined in terms of the brain physiology altered by surgical treatment. We cannot control for the difference the hospital environment makes in patient behavior in contrast with other environments. And we cannot say with precision what a patient would be like if he were not sick; therefore, except for gross forms of behavior, we cannot tell when we have made him well.

Once the surgical lesion is made, it cannot be undone. The brain is thus permanently altered. However one interprets the hypothesis that the brain is the seat of personality, small alterations of the brain can make large differences in behavior. The possibilities of cure and damage are dramatic, though not necessarily immediate. Our concern about psychosurgery as an experimental therapy is dramatically heightened because it is drastic and irreversible. The result is that it needs special consideration as a therapy.

It is possible to dispute this assessment. There is no specific point of transformation of a procedure from "experimental" to "standard." Rather, an innovation moves along a continuum of judgments that bring to bear increasing amounts of information and experience. Despite the opinions of individuals, there does not seem to be a consensus among either the medical community or the public that psychosurgery should be considered standard clinical practice.

The Possibility of Social Abuse

Psychosurgery shares with other new modes of behavior control the promise or the threat of allowing small groups of people to control large groups of other people. The urgency of the matter stems partly from the rapidly increasing sophistication of behavior control techniques; partly from our recent history of social unrest; and partly from the character of the American social structure. In a society in which wealth and power are so unequally distributed, and in which race, ethnicity, and class are as confounded as they are in America, groups which are relatively powerless and easily identifiable, along with others concerned about the protection of individual rights and political dissent, easily perceive the potential threat that psychosurgery could be used for purposes of social control in a medical, therapeutic disguise. From this perspective, psychosurgery is threatening whether it is dangerous or safe, effective or not. There is public concern to protect patients both from insufficiently proven medicine and from procedures employed unnecessarily or out of politically biased definitions of abnormal or antisocial behavior.

Psychosurgery does not lend itself technically to the same wide-scale use as drugs, but in the case of captive populations in the prison and the mental hospital the concern is real and immediate. In these situations psychosurgery could be threatened as a punishment or proferred as a way out of captivity. It might be assented to by a patient because it seems comparatively less destructive than long-term imprisonment or involuntary commitment; it may be just that, under certain circumstances. Possibly the danger lies in constriction of the range of choice open to a prospective patient. As total institutions, prisons and mental hospitals are in themselves coercive in many ways, and certainly they deprive patient candidates of many of the means of protecting themselves which are available to private patients.[2] Regulations for psychosurgery surely must take account of the institutional settings in which the procedures are employed and the civil status of the patient.

The problem posed for developing regulations is how to integrate and balance the therapeutic perspective with the concerns of those who emphasize social influences and consequences. This cannot be done simply by including lawyers and sociologists in committees that prepare guidelines or laws. To do so might only obscure the real conceptual and political problems of integration. Therapeutically oriented people—clinicians, biological researchers, administrators of health-care facilities—tend to ask the following kinds of value questions about their procedures: How efficiently do the procedures accomplish their target goals? What are the side effects? How does a procedure compare with alternative treatments? Or, more philosophically, they might ask what is the justification of the therapeutic goal? Who should set these goals? What is the role of patient consent?

Those more oriented to a social perspective would ask different kinds of questions. What are the social consequences of adopting a certain treatment modality? How would the accepted practice of psychosurgery in prisons alter the means deemed legitimate to maintain institutional order and to protect society? How does the

179

economics of psychosurgery, in contrast to psychoanalysis or behavior modification therapy, tend to preselect patient candidates? How would the social status of the therapist affect his diagnosis, treatment decisions, and postoperative evaluation of different social categories of patients?

Although both groups would acknowledge that the questions of the other are real, each would tend to see the other's concerns as peripheral to the central issues. How can regulations reflect both perspectives, as well as others? If we wait for the emergence of a broader consensus or a higher theoretical perspective, we shall have to wait too long. For the present, we can hope to structure the public discussion of psychosurgery and the deliberations of any regulatory or policy-making body, so that each group comes to appreciate the other's perspective. Each must see its own position as a limited perspective, one among others; the common knowledge of all participants must include the fact that the very nature of the psychosurgery problem depends on the perspective used to interpret it. An adversary model in this case will probably yield the most fruitful results. Rather than decry a situation in which an objective, value-free assessment of facts seems impossible, we might profit by our understanding that the choice of the relevant facts, and our interpretations of them, are at the heart of the controversy. It remains for us to consider those groups to whom regulations or guidelines should be addressed.

Applying Regulations

Words like "regulation," "control," "guidelines," or "review" quite naturally evoke discomfort and even hostility among those who may be the objects of such ministrations, since they understand correctly that their freedom of action is to be constrained to some degree. It would be a mistake, however, to fail to recognize the dual purpose of regulating psychosurgery. Regulations ought to encourage good practice as well as inhibit the bad. What should be encouraged is, first, careful experimentation under controlled conditions in order to establish the therapeutic usefulness of psychosurgical procedures; and, second, the development of a delivery system allowing those who would benefit from its therapy to receive psychosurgery in contexts not threatening to their rights or integrity. What should be proscribed is the practice of psychosurgery where it is not a wise therapy, where it is likely to be abused for nontherapeutic purposes, or where it is used without adequate consent by the patient.

The type of regulations and who is to be regulated are closely related issues. Control mechanisms may be highly informal or strictly codified.[5] Informally, they may include the clinical investigator's conception of his own role and of his criteria for experimentation; professional conferences and staff meetings; journal articles; pressures of the physician-patient relationship; or the influence of the mass media. Formal mechanisms include peer review committees; professional standards of practice; hospital policy; a variety of legal controls, including licensing requirements, malpractice statutes, and court decisions; the rules of federal regulatory agencies; and the funding mechanisms of agencies sponsoring research. Several of these mechanisms have recently been brought into play, including the establishment of review committees at the state level, judicial decisions, funding policies and, most recently, the establishment by Congress of the National Commission for the Protection of Human Subjects of Biomedical and Behavioral Research. This commission's tasks will include the formulation within the next two years of a policy on psychosurgery.

There have already been attempts made to draft regulatory legislation in the Congress. Consider Representative Stokes' bill "to prohibit psychosurgery in federally connected health care facilities."[9] The main features of this bill prohibit persons and institutions from receiving federal money if they perform or allow psychosurgery; make psychosurgery illegal in institutions receiving federal money; provide legal remedies against psychosurgery in terms of civil actions brought by patients or the government; and establish a commission to investigate whether psychosurgery is taking place and what penalties should be levied against those practicing it. The groups addressed include funding agencies and institutions receiving federal funds, members of the commission

181

and those who establish the commission, lawyers for private patients who might bring damage suits, the judiciary, and perhaps indirectly some psychiatrists and neurosurgeons. The guidelines are not addressed directly to psychiatrists and neurosurgeons who might want to know about the effectiveness of various procedures for therapeutic purposes. Indeed, the mechanisms and rationale of the Stokes bill are not made functions of the therapeutic usefulness or social liabilities of psychosurgery at all.

Two difficulties with the bill indicate the problem of addressing regulations to the right groups. In the first place, by effectively preventing psychosurgery by those surgeons and hospital centers geared to careful and systematic research (that research which depends on federal money), the bill would encourage psychosurgery by neurosurgeons unconnected with the large university medical centers, in hospitals and facilities too small to provide the necessary coverage of clinical diagnosis and evaluation, and outside the general public scrutiny given to facilities floating on ponds of federal funds. This is just the opposite of the result that should be sought. If psychosurgery is worthwhile anywhere, it should be performed by surgeons in those contexts best prepared to deal cautiously and carefully with its experimental character.

In the second place, an outright ban on all psychosurgery, even if limited to federally supported contexts, is insensitive to the dual function of regulations. The ability of guidelines both to push and pull depends principally on the issues of therapeutic usefulness and social dangers. It is far better to set conditions under which psychosurgery is permissible rather than simply to ban it. Therefore, the first group to whom regulations should be addressed includes those who conduct clinical investigations. Clinical investigators should be guided to discover, collate, report, and keep current information about the therapeutic uses and dangers of various psychosurgical procedures. Actually, they should provide information about all experimental brain surgery, according to our definition. This information is needed by clinicians and also by the public and its representatives who might circumscribe the use of such therapies over and above the clinician's judgment. A second kind of research that should be guided is that investigating the social context and consequences of psychosurgery. Here we need information about the ways in which psychosurgery might be socially abused and about the means to minimize these dangers. Should psychosurgery become a standard therapy, with proper safeguards against abuse, it may then be possible to protect the rights to treatment of prisoners and other vulnerable groups.

The second major group to be addressed includes clinicians and administrators of health-care facilities, and indirectly the judicial system concerned with issues of malpractice. The objective here is to ensure that diagnosis, treatment, and evaluation of patients reflect judgments based on the results of research, and that hospital protocols provide appropriate interspecialty cooperation and review, including due regard for informed consent. Any experimental neurosurgical procedure should be subject to careful professional and institutional protocols.

The third major group includes administrators of institutions such as prisons and mental hospitals which house captive populations. Here the social status of the patient must be weighed most carefully against his medical status. Special consideration must be given to the ability of the patient to consent within a context that is inherently coercive and in which the dangers of misdiagnosis are greater than usual. These regulations would thus emphasize the special difficulties arising from the institutional settings in which surgery would take place. Questions of motive will inevitably intrude, and special precautions may have to be taken.

One other group would profit from a knowledge of such regulations, and that includes journalists and others who represent and inform the public on the whole array of experimentation in behavior control. By making public what is happening and by contributing their own interpretations of events and issues, they increase the likelihood that a "medical" process will be subject to public, especially legal, review and control. It is to everyone's benefit to have accurate and complete information when assessing these practices.

The actual drafting of regulations for psychosurgery, and the choice of appropriate models, will be a complex matter. My purpose has been to indicate the nature of the issues involved in regulation and to illuminate certain major areas of concern to those who will write guidelines or draft regulatory policies.

REFERENCES

1. Falconer, M. "Reversibility by Temporal-Lobe Resection of the Behavioral Abnormalities of Temporal Lobe Epilepsy." *New England Journal of Medicine*, 289(1973): 451-455.

2. Goffman, E. *Asylums: Essays on the Social Situation of Mental Patients and Other Inmates.* Garden City, L.I., N.Y.: Doubleday (Anchor Books), 1961.

3. Goldstein, M. "Brain Research and Violent Behavior. A Summary and Evaluation of the Status of Biomedical Research on Brain and Aggressive Violent Behavior." *Archives of Neurology*, 30(1974): 1-35.

4. Hitchcock, E., Laitinen, L., and Vaernet, K., eds. *Psychosurgery.* Springfield, Ill.: Charles C. Thomas, 1972.

5. Klerman, G., Neville, R., and Swazey, J. "Regulatory Models for Therapeutic Innovation: Surgery and Drugs." Unpublished manuscript prepared for the Behavior Control Project of the Institute of Society, Ethics, and the Life Sciences, New York.

6. Mark, V., and Neville, R. "Social and Ethical Implications of Brain Surgery in Aggressive Epileptics." *Journal of the American Medical Association* 226(1973): 765-772.

7. "Relieving Intractable Pain Remains a Problem for Physicians." *Journal of the American Medical Association* 225(1973): 9-13.

8. Sedgwick, P. "Illness—Mental and Otherwise." *Hastings Center Studies* 1 (1973): 19-40.

9. Stokes, Rep. L. H.R. 6852, 93rd Cong., 1st sess., introduced April 11, 1973.

10. Ström-Olsen, R. and Carlisle, S. "Bi-Frontal Stereotactic Tractotomy." *British Journal of Psychiatry* 118(1971): 141-154.

11. Szasz, T. *The Myth of Mental Illness.* New York: Dell, 1961.

12. _____ . *The Manufacture of Madness.* New York: Dell, 1970.

Appendix

STATE OF MICHIGAN

IN THE CIRCUIT COURT FOR THE COUNTY OF WAYNE

GABE KAIMOWITZ, representing himself)
and certain individual members of the)
Medical Committee for Human Rights)
on behalf of)
)
JOHN DOE and at least 23 others)
similarly situated who are held or)
committed involuntarily in public)
institutions in Michigan,)
) CIVIL ACTION
              Petitioners - Plaintiffs,) NO. 73-19434-AW
and)
)
JOHN DOE,)
              Intervenor - Plaintiff,)
-VS-)
)
DEPARTMENT OF MENTAL HEALTH FOR THE)
STATE OF MICHIGAN, DR. E. G. YUDASHKIN,)
Director, State Department of Mental)
Health; DR. J. S. GOTTLIEB, Director)
Lafayette Clinic; DR. ERNST RODIN,)
Associate of Dr. Gottlieb at the Clinic,)
in their official capacities, as well as)
their agents, assignees, employees, and)
successors in office,)
)
              Respondents - Defendants,)
)
AMERICAN ORTHOPSYCHIATRIC ASSOCIATION,)
)
              Amicus Curiae.)
)
                   -)

OPINION

This case came to this Court originally on a complaint for a Writ of Habeas Corpus brought by Plaintiff Kaimowitz on behalf of John Doe and the Medical Committee for Human Rights, alleging that John Doe was being illegally detained in the Lafayette Clinic for the purpose of experimental psychosurgery.[1]

John Doe had been committed by the Kalamazoo County Circuit Court on January 11, 1955, to the Ionia State Hospital as a Criminal Sexual Psycho-

---

[1]The name John Doe has been used through the proceedings to protect the true identity of the subject involved. After the institution of this action and during proceedings his true identity was revealed. His true name is Louis Smith. For the purpose of the Opinion, however, he will be referred to throughout as John Doe.

APPENDIX

path, without a trial of criminal charges, under the terms of the then existing Criminal Sexual Psychopathic law.[2] He had been charged with the murder and subsequent rape of a student nurse at the Kalamazoo State Hospital while he was confined there as a mental patient.

In 1972, Drs. Ernst Rodin and Jacques Gottlieb of the Lafayette Clinic, a facility of the Michigan Department of Mental Health, had filed a proposal "For the Study of Treatment of Uncontrollable Aggression."[3]

This was funded by the Legislature of the State of Michigan for the fiscal year 1972. After more than 17 years at the Ionia State Hospital, John Doe was transferred to the Lafayette Clinic in November of 1972 as a suitable research subject for the Clinic's study of uncontrollable aggression.

Under the terms of the study, 24 criminal sexual psychopaths in the State's mental health system were to be subjects of experiment. The experiment was to compare the effects of surgery on the amygdaloid portion of the limbic system of the brain with the effect of the drug cyproterone acetate on the male hormone flow. The comparison was intended to show which, if either, could be used in controlling aggression of males in an institutional setting, and to afford lasting permanent relief from such aggression to the patient.

Substantial difficulties were encountered in locating a suitable patient population for the surgical procedures and a matched controlled group for the treatment by the anti-androgen drug.[4] As a matter of fact, it was concluded that John Doe was the only known appropriate candidate available within the state mental health system for the surgical experiment.

John Doe signed an "informed consent" form to become an experimental subject prior to his transfer from the Ionia State Hospital.[5] He had obtained signatures from his parents giving consent for the experimental

---

[2]C.L. 780.501 et seq. The statute under which he was committed was repealed by Public Act 143 of the Public Acts of 1968, effective August 1, 1968. He was detained thereafter under C.L. 330.35 (b), which provided for further detention and release of criminal sexual psychopaths under the repealed statute. The Supreme Court also adopted an Administrative Order of October 20, 1969 (382 Mich. xxix) relating to criminal sexual psychopaths. A full discussion of these statutes is found in the Court's earlier Opinion relating to the legality of detention of John Doe, filed in this cause on March 23, 1973.

[3]See Appendix to Opinion, Item 1.

[4]For criteria, see Appendix, Item 2.

[5]The complete "Informed Consent" form signed by John Doe is as follows:

"Since conventional treatment efforts over a period of several years have not enabled me to control my outbursts of rage and anti-social behavior, I submit an application to be a subject in a research project which may offer me a form of effective therapy. This therapy is based upon the idea that episodes of anti-social rage and sexuality might be triggered by a disturbance in certain portions of my brain. I understand that in order to be certain that a significant brain disturbance exists, which might relate to my anti-social behavior, an initial operation will have to be performed. This procedure consists of placing fine wires into my brain, which will record the electrical activity from those structures which play a part in anger and sexuality. These electrical waves can then be studied to determine the presence of an abnormality.

186

and innovative surgical procedures to be performed on his brain,[6] and two separate three-man review committees were established by Dr. Rodin to review the scientific worthiness of the study and the validity of the consent obtained from Doe.

The Scientific Review Committee, headed by Dr. Elliot Luby, approved of the procedure, and the Human Rights Review Committee, consisting of Ralph Slovenko, a Professor of Law and Psychiatry at Wayne State University, Monsignor Clifford Sawher, and Frank Moran, a Certified Public Accountant, gave their approval to the procedure.

Even though no experimental subjects were found to be available in the state mental health system other than John Doe, Dr. Rodin prepared to proceed with the experiment on Doe, and depth electrodes were to be inserted into his brain on or about January 15, 1973.

Early in January, 1973, Plaintiff Kaimowitz became aware of the work being contemplated on John Doe and made his concern known to the Detroit Free Press. Considerable newspaper publicity ensued and this action was filed shortly thereafter.

With the rush of publicity on the filing of the original suit, funds for the research project were stopped by Dr. Gordon Yudashkin, Director of the Department of Mental Health, and the investigators, Drs. Gottlieb and Rodin, dropped their plans to pursue the research set out in the proposal. They reaffirmed at trial, however, their belief in the scientific, medical and ethical soundness of the proposal.

"In addition electrical stimulation with weak currents passed through these wires will be done in order to find out if one or several points in the brain can trigger my episodes of violence or unlawful sexuality. In other words this stimulation may cause me to want to commit an aggressive or sexual act, but every effort will be made to have a sufficient number of people present to control me. If the brain disturbance is limited to a small area, I understand that the investigators will destroy this part of my brain with an electrical current. If the abnormality comes from a larger part of my brain, I agree that it should be surgically removed, if the doctors determine that it can be done so, without risk of side effects. Should the electrical activity from the parts of my brain into which the wires have been placed reveal that there is no significant abnormality, the wires will simply be withdrawn.

"I realize that any operation on the brain carries a number of risks which may be slight, but could be potentially serious. These risks include infection, bleeding, temporary or permanent weakness or paralysis of one or more of my legs or arms, difficulties with speech and thinking, as well as the ability to feel, touch, pain and temperature. Under extraordinary circumstances, it is also possible that I might not survive the operation.

"Fully aware of the risks detailed in the paragraphs above, I authorize the physicians of Lafayette Clinic and Providence Hospital to perform the procedures as outlined above.

October 27, 1972	/S/ Louis M. Smith
Date	Signature

Calvin Vanee	/S/ Emily T. Smith/Harry L. Smith
Witness	Signature of responsible relative or guardian

---

[6]There is some dispute in the record as to whether his parents gave consent for the innovative surgical procedures. They testified they gave consent only to the insertion of depth electrodes.

187

APPENDIX

Upon the request of counsel, a Three-Judge Court was empanelled, Judges John D. O'Hair and George E. Bowles joining Judge Horace W. Gilmore. Dean Francis A. Allen and Prof. Robert A. Burt of the University of Michigan Law School were appointed as counsel for John Doe.

Approximately the same time Amicus Curiae, the American Orthopsychiatric Society, sought to enter the case with the right to offer testimony. This was granted by the Court.

Three ultimate issues were framed for consideration by the Court. The first related to the constitutionality of the detention of Doe. The full statement of the second and third questions, to which this Opinion is addressed, are set forth in the text below.

The first issue relating to the constitutionality of the detention of John Doe was considered by the Court, and on March 23, 1973, an Opinion was rendered by the Court holding the detention unconstitutional. Subsequently, after hearing testimony of John Doe's present condition, the Court directed his release.[7]

In the meantime, since it appeared unlikely that any project would go forward because of the withdrawal of approval by Dr. Yudashkin, the Court raised the question as to whether the rest of the case had become moot. All counsel, except counsel representing the Department of Mental Health, stated the matter was not moot, and that the basic issues involved were ripe for declaratory judgment. Counsel for the Department of Mental Health contended the matter was moot.

Full argument was had and the Court on March 15, 1973, rendered an oral Opinion, holding that the matter was not moot and that the case should proceed as to the two framed issues for declaratory judgment. The Court held that even though the original experimental program was terminated, there was nothing that would prevent it from being instituted again in the near future, and therefore the matter was ripe for declaratory judgment.[8]

---

[7]The release was directed after the testimony of John Doe in open court and the testimony of Dr. Andrew S. Watson, who felt that John Doe could be safely released to society.

[8]On Thursday, March 15, 1973, after full argument, the Court held in an Opinion rendered from the bench that the matter was not moot, relying upon United States v. Phosphate Export Association, 393 U. S. 199. There the United States Supreme Court said:

> "The test for mootness . . . is a stringent one. Mere voluntary cessation of allegedly illegal conduct does not moot a case; if it did, the courts would be compelled to 'leave the defendant . . . free to return to his old ways.' A case might become moot if subsequent events made it absolutely clear that the allegedly wrongful behavior could not reasonably be expected to recur."

The Court also relied upon Milford v. Peoples Community Hospital Authority, 380 Mich. 49, where the Court said on page 55:

> "The nature of the case is such that we are unlikely to again receive the question in the near future, and doctors and other people dealing with public hospital corporations cannot

The facts concerning the original experiment and the involvement of John Doe were to be considered by the Court as illustrative in determining whether legally adequate consent could be obtained from adults involuntarily confined in the state mental health system for experimental or innovative procedures on the brain to ameliorate behavior, and, if it could be, whether the State should allow such experimentation on human subjects to proceed.[9]

The two issues framed for decision in this declaratory judgment action are as follows:

1. After failure of established therapies, may an adult or a legally appointed guardian, if the adult is involuntarily detained, at a facility within the jurisdiction of the State Department of Mental Health give legally adequate consent to an innovative or experimental surgical procedure on the brain, if there is demonstrable physical abnormality of the brain, and the procedure is designed to ameliorate behavior, which is either personally tormenting to the patient, or so profoundly disruptive that the patient cannot safely live, or live with others?

2. If the answer to the above is yes, then is it legal in this State to undertake an innovative or experimental surgical procedure on the brain of an adult who is involuntarily detained at a facility within the jurisdiction of the State Department of Mental Health, if there is demonstrable physical abnormality of the brain, and the procedure is designed to ameliorate behavior, which is either personally tormenting to the patient, or so profoundly disruptive that the patient cannot safely live, or live with others?

Throughout this Opinion, the Court will use the term psychosurgery to describe the proposed innovative or experimental surgical procedure defined in the questions for consideration by the Court.

At least two definitions of psychosurgery have been furnished the Court. Dr. Bertram S. Brown, Director of the National Institute of Mental Health, defined the term as follows in his prepared statement before the United States Senate Subcommittee on Health of the Committee on Labor and Public Welfare on February 23, 1973:

> "Psychosurgery can best be defined as a surgical removal or destruction of brain tissue or the cutting of brain tissue to disconnect one part of the brain from another, with the intent of altering the behavior, even though there may be no direct evidence of structural disease or damage to the brain."

---

hope to have an answer to the questions raised unless we proceed to decision. For these reasons, we conclude the case is of sufficient importance to warrant our decision."

It should also be noted that Defendant Department of Mental Health sought an Order of Superintending Control for a Stay of Proceedings in the Court of Appeals on the ground the case was moot. On March 26, 1973, the Court of Appeals denied the Stay.

[9]As the trial proceeded, it was learned that John Doe himself withdrew his consent to such experimentation. This still did not render the proceeding moot because of the questions framed for declaratory judgment.

APPENDIX

Dr. Peter Breggin, a witness at the trial, defined psychosurgery as the destruction of normal brain tissue for the control of emotions or behavior; or the destruction of abnormal brain tissue for the control of emotions or behavior, where the abnormal tissue has not been shown to be the cause of the emotions or behavior in question.

The psychosurgery involved in this litigation is a subclass, narrower than that defined by Dr. Brown. The proposed psychosurgery we are concerned with encompasses only experimental psychosurgery where there are demonstrable physical abnormalities in the brain.[10] Therefore, temporal lobectomy, an established therapy for relief of clearly diagnosed epilepsy is not involved, nor are accepted neurological surgical procedures, for example, operations for Parkinsonism, or operations for the removal of tumors or the relief of stroke.

We start with the indisputable medical fact that no significant activity in the brain occurs in isolation without correlated activity in other parts of the brain. As the level of complexity of human behavior increases, so does the degree of interaction and integration. Dr. Ayub Ommaya, a witness in the case, illustrated this through the phenomenon of vision. Pure visual sensation is one of the functions highly localized in the occipital lobe in the back of the brain. However, vision in its broader sense, such as the ability to recognize a face, does not depend upon this area of the brain alone. It requires the integration of that small part of the brain with the rest of the brain. Memory mechanisms interact with the visual sensation to permit the recognition of the face. Dr. Ommaya pointed out that the more we know about brain function, the more we realize with certainty that many functions are highly integrated, even for relatively simple activity.

It is clear from the record in this case that the understanding of the limbic system of the brain and its function is very limited. Practically every witness and exhibit established how little is known of the relationship of the limbic system to human behavior, in the absence of some clearly defined clinical disease such as epilepsy. Drs. Mark, Sweet and Ervin have noted repeatedly the primitive state of our understanding of the amygdala, for example, remarking that it is an area made up of nine to fourteen different nuclear structures, with many functions, some of which

---

[10]On this point, Amicus Curiae Exhibit 4 is of great interest. This exhibit is a memo to Dr. Gottlieb from Dr. Rodin, dated August 9, 1972, reporting on a visit Dr. Rodin made to Dr. Vernon H. Mark of the Neurological Research Foundation in Boston, one of the country's leading proponents of psychosurgery on noninstitutionalized patients. Dr. Rodin, in his Memo, stated:

"When I informed Dr. Mark of our project, namely, doing amygdalotomies on patients who do not have epilepsy, he became extremely concerned and stated, we had no ethical right in so doing. This, of course, opened Pandora's box, because then I retorted that he was misleading us with his previously cited book and he had no right at all from a scientific point of view to state that in the human, aggression is accompanied by seizure discharges in the amygdala, because he is dealing with only patients who have susceptible brains, namely, temporal lobe epilepsy. . . ."

"He stated categorically that as far as present evidence is concerned, one has no right to make lesions in a 'healthy brain' when the individual suffers from rage attacks only."

190

are competitive with others. They state that there are not even reliable guesses as to the functional location of some of the nuclei.[11]

The testimony showed that any physical intervention in the brain must always be approached with extreme caution. Brain surgery is always irreversible in the sense that any intrusion into the brain destroys the brain cells and such cells do not regenerate. Dr. Ommaya testified that in the absence of well-defined pathological signs, such as blood clots pressing on the brain due to trauma, or tumor in the brain, brain surgery is viewed as a treatment of last resort.

The record in this case demonstrates that animal experimentation and non-intrusive human experimentation have not been exhausted in determining and studying brain function. Any experimentation on the human brain, especially when it involves an intrusive, irreversible procedure in a non-life-threatening situation, should be undertaken with extreme caution, and then only when answers cannot be obtained from animal experimentation and from non-intrusive human experimentation.

Psychosurgery should never be undertaken upon involuntarily committed populations, when there is a high-risk low-benefit ratio as demonstrated in this case. This is because of the impossibility of obtaining truly informed consent from such populations. The reasons such informed consent cannot be obtained are set forth in detail subsequently in this Opinion.

There is widespread concern about violence. Personal violence, whether in a domestic setting or reflected in street violence, tends to increase. Violence in group confrontations appears to have culminated in the late 60's but still invites study and suggested solutions. Violence, personal and group, has engaged the criminal law courts and the correctional systems, and has inspired the appointment of national commissions. The late President Lyndon B. Johnson convened a commission on violence under the chairmanship of Dr. Milton Eisenhower. It was a commission that had fifty consultants representing various fields of law, sociology, criminology, history, government, social psychiatry, and social psychology. Conspicuous by their absence were any professionals concerned with the human brain. It is not surprising, then, that of recent date, there has been theorizing as to violence and the brain, and just over two years ago, Frank Ervin, a psychiatrist, and Vernon H. Mark, a neurosurgeon, wrote Violence and the Brain[12] detailing the application of brain surgery to problems of violent behavior.

Problems of violence are not strangers to this Court. Over many years we have studied personal and group violence in a court context. Nor are we unconcerned about the tragedies growing out of personal or group confrontations. Deep-seated public concern begets an impatient desire for miracle solutions. And necessarily, we deal here not only with legal and medical issues, but with ethical and social issues as well.

Is brain function related to abnormal aggressive behavior? This, fundamentally, is what the case is about. But, one cannot segment or simplify that which is inherently complex. As Vernon H. Mark has written, "Moral values are social concerns, not medical ones, in any presently recognized sense."[13]

---

[11]Mark, Sweet and Ervin, "The Affect of Amygdalotomy on Violent Behavior in Patients with Temporal Lobe Epilepsy," in Hitchcock, Ed. Psycho-Surgery: Second International Conference (Thomas Pub. 1972), 135 at 153.

[12]Mark and Ervin, Violence and the Brain (Harper & Row, 1970).

[13]Mark, "Brain Surgery in Aggressive Epileptics," the Hastings Center Report, Vol. 3, No. 1 (February, 1973).

APPENDIX

Violent behavior not associated with brain disease should not be dealt with surgically. At best, neurosurgery rightfully should concern itself with medical problems and not the behavior problems of a social etiology.

The Court does not in any way desire to impede medical progress. We are much concerned with violence and the possible effect of brain disease on violence. Much research on the brain is necessary and must be carried on, but when it takes the form of psychosurgery, it cannot be undertaken on involuntarily detained populations. Other avenues of research must be utilized and developed.

Although extensive psychosurgery has been performed in the United States and throughout the world in recent years to attempt change of objectionable behavior, there is no medically recognized syndrome for aggression and objectionable behavior associated with nonorganic brain abnormality.

The psychosurgery that has been done has in varying degrees blunted emotions and reduced spontaneous behavior. Dr. V. Balasubramaniam, a leading psychosurgeon, has characterized psychosurgery as "sedative neuro-surgery," a procedure by which patients are made quiet and manageable.[14] The amygdalotomy, for example, has been used to calm hyperactive children, to make retarded children more manageable in institutions, to blunt the emotions of people with depression, and to attempt to make schizophrenics more manageable.[15]

As pointed out above, psychosurgery is clearly experimental, poses substantial danger to research subjects, and carries substantial unknown risks. There is no persuasive showing on this record that the type of psychosurgery we are concerned with would necessarily confer any sub-stantial benefit on research subjects or significantly increase the body of scientific knowledge by providing answers to problems of deviant behavior.

The dangers of such surgery are undisputed. Though it may be urged, as

---

[14]See Defendant's Exhibit 38, "Sedative Neurosurgery" by V. Balasubramaniam, T. S. Kanaka, P. V. Ramanuman, and B. Ramaurthi, 53 Journal of the Indian Medical Association, No. 8, page 377 (1969). In the conclusion, page 381, the writer said:

"The main purpose of this communication is to show that this new form of surgery called sedative neurosurgery is available for the treatment of certain groups of disorders. These disorders are primarily characterized by restlessness, low threshold for anger and violent or destructive tendencies.

"This operation aims at destruction of certain areas in the brain. These targets include the amygdaloid nuclei, the postero-ventral nuclear group of the hypothalamus and the periaqueductal grey substance. . . ."

"By operating on the areas one can make these patients quiet and manageable."

[15]The classical lobotomy of which thousands were performed in the 1940's and 1950's is very rarely used these days. The development of drug therapy pretty well did away with the classical lobotomy. Follow-up studies show that the lobotomy procedure was overused and caused a great deal of damage to the persons who were subjected to it. A general bleaching of the personality occurred and the operations were associated with loss of drive and concentration. Dr. Brown in his testimony before the United States Senate, supra, page 9, stated: "No responsible scientist today would condone a classical lobotomy operation."

192

did some of the witnesses in this case, that the incidents of morbidity and mortality are low from the procedures, all agree dangers are involved, and the benefits to the patient are uncertain.

Absent a clearly defined medical syndrome, nothing pinpoints the exact location in the brain of the cause of undesirable behavior so as to enable a surgeon to make a lesion, remove that portion of the brain, and thus affect undesirable behavior.

Psychosurgery flattens emotional responses, leads to lack of abstract reasoning ability, leads to a loss of capacity for new learning and causes general sedation and apathy. It can lead to impairment of memory, and in some instances unexpected responses to psychosurgery are observed. It has been found, for example, that heightened rage reaction can follow surgical intervention on the amygdala, just as placidity can.[16]

It was unanimously agreed by all witnesses that psychosurgery does not, given the present state of the art, provide any assurance that a dangerously violent person can be restored to the community.[17]

Simply stated, on this record there is no scientific basis for establishing that the removal or destruction of an area of the limbic brain would have any direct therapeutic effect in controlling aggressivity or improving tormenting personal behavior, absent the showing of a well-defined clinical syndrome such as epilepsy.

To advance scientific knowledge, it is true that doctors may desire to experiment on human beings, but the need for scientific inquiry must be reconciled with the inviolability which our society provides for a person's mind and body. Under a free government, one of a person's greatest rights is the right to inviolability of his person, and it is axiomatic that this right necessarily forbids the physician or surgeon from violating, without permission, the bodily integrity of his patient.[18]

Generally, individuals are allowed free choice about whether to undergo experimental medical procedures. But the State has the power to modify this free choice concerning experimental medical procedures when it cannot be freely given, or when the result would be contrary to public policy. For example, it is obvious that a person may not consent to acts that will constitute murder, manslaughter, or mayhem upon himself.[19] In short, there are times when the State for good reason should withhold a person's ability to consent to certain medical procedures.

It is elementary tort law that consent is the mechanism by which the patient grants the physician the power to act, and which protects the

---

[16]Sweet, Mark & Ervin found this to be true in experiments with monkeys. Other evidence indicated it is possible in human beings.

[17]Testimony in the case from Dr. Rodin, Dr. Lowinger, Dr. Breggin, and Dr. Walter, all pointed up that it is very difficult to find the risks, deficits and benefits from psychosurgery because of the failure of the literature to provide adequate research information about research subjects before and after surgery.

[18]See the language of the late Justice Cardozo in Schloendorff v. Society of New York Hospitals, 211 N. Y. 125, 105 N. E. 92, 93 (1914) where he said, "Every human being of adult years or sound mind has a right to determine what shall be done with his own body. . . ."

[19]See "Experimentation on Human Beings," 22 Stanford Law Review 99 (1967); Kidd, "Limits of the Right of a Person to Consent to Experimentation Upon Himself," 117 Science 211 (1953).

patient against unauthorized invasions of his person. This requirement
protects one of society's most fundamental values, the inviolability of
the individual. An operation performed upon a patient without his informed
consent is the tort of battery, and a doctor and a hospital have no right
to impose compulsory medical treatment against the patient's will. These
elementary statements of tort law need no citation.

Jay Katz, in his outstanding book Experimentation with Human Beings
(Russell Sage Foundation, N.Y. (1972)) points out on page 523 that the
concept of informed consent has been accepted as a cardinal principle for
judging the propriety of research with human beings.

He points out that in the experimental setting, informed consent
serves multiple purposes. He states (pages 523 and 524):

". . . Most clearly, requiring informed consent serves
society's desire to respect each individual's autonomy, and his
right to make choices concerning his own life.

"Second, providing a subject with information about an
experiment will encourage him to be an active partner and the
process may also increase the rationality of the experimentation
process.

"Third, securing informed consent protects the experimentation process by encouraging the investigator to question the value
of the proposed project and the adequacy of the measures he has
taken to protect subjects, by reducing civil and criminal liability
for nonnegligent injury to the subjects, and by diminishing adverse
public reaction to an experiment.

"Finally, informed consent may serve the function of increasing society's awareness about human research. . . ."

It is obvious that there must be close scrutiny of the adequacy of the
consent when an experiment, as in this case, is dangerous, intrusive,
irreversible, and of uncertain benefit to the patient and society.[20]

Counsel for Drs. Rodin and Gottlieb argues that anyone who has ever
been treated by a doctor for any relatively serious illness is likely to
acknowledge that a competent doctor can get almost any patient to consent
to almost anything. Counsel claims this is true because patients do not
want to make decisions about complex medical matters and because there is
the general problem of avoiding decision making in stress situations,
characteristic of all human beings.

He further argues that a patient is always under duress when hospitalized and that in a hospital or institutional setting there is no such
thing as a volunteer. Dr. Ingelfinger in Volume 287, page 466, of the New
England Journal of Medicine (August 31, 1972) states:

---

[20]The principle is reflected in numerous statements of medical ethics.
See the American Medical Association, "Principles of Medical Ethics," 132
JAMA 1090 (1946); American Medical Association, "Ethical Guidelines for
Clinical Investigation" (1966); National Institute of World Medical Association, "Code of Ethics" (Declaration of Helsinki) reprinted in 2
British Medical Journal, 177 (1964). It is manifested in the code adopted
by the United States Military Tribunal at Nuremberg which, at the time,
was considered the most carefully developed precept specifically drawn to
meet the problems of human experimentation. See Ladimer, I. "Ethical and
Legal Aspects of Medical Research in Human Beings," 3 J. Pub. L. 467, 487
(1954).

". . . The process of obtaining 'informed consent' with all its regulations and conditions, is no more than an elaborate ritual, a device that when the subject is uneducated and uncomprehending, confers no more than the semblance of propriety on human experimentation. The subject's only real protection, the public as well as the medical profession must recognize, depends on the conscience and compassion of the investigator and his peers."

Everything defendants' counsel argues militates against the obtaining of informed consent from involuntarily detained mental patients. If, as he argues, truly informed consent cannot be given for regular surgical procedures by noninstitutionalized persons, then certainly an adequate informed consent cannot be given by the involuntarily detained mental patient.

We do not agree that a truly informed consent cannot be given for a regular surgical procedure by a patient, institutionalized or not. The law has long recognized that such valid consent can be given. But we do hold that informed consent cannot be given by an involuntarily detained mental patient for experimental psychosurgery for the reasons set forth below.

The Michigan Supreme Court has considered in a tort case the problems of experimentation with humans. In Hortner v. Koch, 272 Mich. 273, 261 N. W. 762 (1935), the issue turned on whether the doctor had taken proper diagnostic steps before prescribing an experimental treatment for cancer. Discussing medical experimentation, the Court said at page 282:

"We recognize the fact that if the general practice of medicine and surgery is to progress, there must be a certain amount of experimentation carried on; but such experiments must be done with the knowledge and consent of the patient or those responsible for him, and must not vary too radically from the accepted method of procedure. (Emphasis added).

This means that the physician cannot experiment without restraint or restriction. He must consider first of all the welfare of his patient. This concept is universally accepted by the medical profession, the legal profession, and responsible persons who have thought and written on the matter.

Furthermore, he must weigh the risk to the patient against the benefit to be obtained by trying something new. The risk-benefit ratio is an important ratio in considering any experimental surgery upon a human being. The risk must always be relatively low, in the non-life-threatening situation to justify human experimentation.

Informed consent is a requirement of variable demands. Being certain that a patient has consented adequately to an operation, for example, is much more important when doctors are going to undertake an experimental, dangerous, and intrusive procedure than, for example, when they are going to remove an appendix. When a procedure is experimental, dangerous, and intrusive, special safeguards are necessary. The risk-benefit ratio must be carefully considered, and the question of consent thoroughly explored.

To be legally adequate, a subject's informed consent must be competent, knowing and voluntary.

In considering consent for experimentation, the ten principles known as the Nuremberg Code give guidance. They are found in the Judgment of the Court in United States v. Karl Brandt.[21]

[21]Trial of War Criminals before the Nuremberg Military Tribunals. Volume 1 and 2, "The Medical Case," Washington, D. C.; U. S. Government Printing Office (1948) reprinted in Experimentation with Human Beings, by Katz (Russell Sage Foundation (1972) page 305.

APPENDIX

There the Court said:

". . . Certain basic principles must be observed in order to satisfy moral, ethical and legal concepts:

1. The voluntary consent of the human subject is absolutely essential.

This means that the person involved should have legal capacity to give consent; should be so situated as to be able to exercise free power of choice, without the intervention of any element of force, fraud, deceit, duress, overreaching, or other ulterior form of constraint or coercion; and should have sufficient knowledge and comprehension of the elements of the subject matter involved as to enable him to make an understanding and enlightened decision. This latter element requires that before the acceptance of an affirmative decision by the experimental subject, there should be made known to him the nature, duration and purpose of the experiment; the methods and means by which it is to be conducted; all inconveniences and hazards reasonably to be expected; and the affects upon his health or person which may possibly come from his participation in the experiment.

The duty and responsibility for ascertaining the quality of the consent rests upon each individual who initiates, directs, or engages in the experiment. It is a personal duty and responsibility which may not be delegated to another with impunity.

"2. The experiment should be such as to yield fruitful results for the good of society, unprocurable by other methods or means of study, and not random and unnecessary in nature.

"3. The experiment should be so designed and based on the results of animal experimentation and a knowledge of the natural history of the disease or other problem under study that the anticipated results will justify the performance of the experiment.

"4. The experiment should be so conducted as to avoid all unnecessary physical and mental suffering and injury.

"5. No experiment should be conducted where there is an a priori reason to believe that death or disabling injury will occur; except, perhaps, in those experiments where the experimental physicians also serve as subjects.

"6. The degree of risk to be taken should never exceed that determined by the humanitarian importance of the problem to be solved by the experiment.

"7. Proper preparations should be made and adequate facilities provided to protect the experimental subject against even remote possibilities of injury, disability, or death.

"8. The experiment should be conducted only by scientifically qualified persons. The highest degree of skill and care should be required through all stages of the experiment of those who conduct or engage in the experiment.

"9. During the course of the experiment the human subject should be at liberty to bring the experiment to an end if he has reached the physical or mental state where continuation of the experiment seems to him to be impossible.

"10. During the course of the experiment the scientist in charge must be prepared to terminate the experiment at any stage, if he has probable cause to believe, in the exercise of the good faith, superior skill,.and careful judgment required of him that a continuation of the experiment is likely to result in injury, disability, or death to the experimental subject."

In the Nuremberg Judgment, the elements of what must guide us in decision are found. The involuntarily detained mental patient must have legal capacity to give consent. He must be so situated as to be able to exercise free power of choice without any element of force, fraud, deceit, duress, overreaching, or other ulterior form of restraint or coercion. He must have sufficient knowledge and comprehension of the subject matter to enable him to make an understanding decision. The decision must be a totally voluntary one on his part.

We must first look to the competency of the involuntarily detained mental patient to consent. Competency requires the ability of the subject to understand rationally the nature of the procedure, its risks, and other relevant information. The standard governing required disclosure by a doctor is what a reasonable patient needs to know in order to make an intelligent decision. See Waltz and Scheunenman, "Informed Consent Therapy," 64 Northwestern Law Review 628 (1969).[22]

Although an involuntarily detained mental patient may have a sufficient I. Q. to intellectually comprehend his circumstances (in Dr. Rodin's experiment, a person was required to have at least an I. Q. of 80), the very nature of his incarceration diminishes the capacity to consent to psychosurgery. He is particularly vulnerable as a result of his mental condition, the deprivation stemming from involuntary confinement, and the effects of the phenomenon of "institutionalization."

The very moving testimony of John Doe in the instant case establishes this beyond any doubt. The fact of institutional confinement has special force in undermining the capacity of the mental patient to make a competent decision on this issue, even though he be intellectually competent to do so. In the routine of institutional life, most decisions are made for patients. For example, John Doe testified how extraordinary it was for him to be approached by Dr. Yudashkin about the possible submission to psychosurgery, and how unusual it was to be consulted by a physician about his preference.

Institutionalization tends to strip the individual of the supports which permit him to maintain his sense of self-worth and the value of his own physical and mental integrity. An involuntarily confined mental patient clearly has diminished capacity for making a decision about irreversible experimental psychosurgery.

Equally great problems are found when the involuntarily detained mental patient is incompetent, and consent is sought from a guardian or parent. Although guardian or parental consent may be legally adequate when arising out of traditional circumstances, it is legally ineffective in the

[22]In Ballentine's Law Dictionary (Second Edition) (1948), competency is equated with capacity and capacity is defined as "a person's ability to understand the nature and effect of the act in which he is engaged and the business in which he is transacting."

psychosurgery situation. The guardian or parent cannot do that which the patient, absent a guardian, would be legally unable to do.

The second element of an informed consent is knowledge of the risk involved and the procedures to be undertaken. It was obvious from the record made in this case that the facts surrounding experimental brain surgery are profoundly uncertain, and the lack of knowledge on the subject makes a knowledgable consent to psychosurgery literally impossible.

We turn now to the third element of an informed consent, that of voluntariness. It is obvious that the most important thing to a large number of involuntarily detained mental patients incarcerated for an unknown length of time, is freedom.

The Nuremberg standards require that the experimental subjects be so situated as to exercise free power of choice without the intervention of any element of force, fraud, deceit, duress, overreaching, or other ulterior form of constraint or coercion. It is impossible for an involuntarily detained mental patient to be free of ulterior forms of restraint or coercion when his very release from the institution may depend upon his cooperating with the institutional authorities and giving consent to experimental surgery.

The privileges of an involuntarily detained patient and the rights he exercises in the institution are within the control of the institutional authorities. As was pointed out in the testimony of John Doe, such minor things as the right to have a lamp in his room, or the right to have ground privileges to go for a picnic with his family assumed major proportions. For 17 years he lived completely under the control of the hospital. Nearly every important aspect of his life was decided without any opportunity on his part to participate in the decision-making process.

The involuntarily detained mental patient is in an inherently coercive atmosphere even though no direct pressures may be placed upon him. He finds himself stripped of customary amenities and defenses. Free movement is restricted. He becomes a part of communal living subject to the control of the institutional authorities.

As pointed out in the testimony in this case, John Doe consented to this psychosurgery partly because of his effort to show the doctors in the hospital that he was a cooperative patient. Even Dr. Yudashkin, in his testimony, pointed out that involuntarily confined patients tend to tell their doctors what the patient thinks these people want to hear.

The inherently coercive atmosphere to which the involuntarily detained mental patient is subjected has bearing upon the voluntariness of his consent. This was pointed up graphically by Dr. Watson in his testimony (page 67, April 4.) There he was asked if there was any significant difference between the kinds of coercion that exist in an open hospital setting and the kinds of coercion that exist on involuntarily detained patients in a state mental institution.

Dr. Watson answered in this way:

"There is an enormous difference. My perception of the patients at Ionia is that they are willing almost to try anything to somehow or other improve their lot, which is--you know-- not bad. It is just plain normal--you know--that kind of desire. Again, that pressure--again--I don't like to use the word 'coercion' because it implies a kind of deliberateness and that is not what we are talking about--the pressure to accede is perhaps the more accurate way, I think--the pressure is perhaps so severe that it probably ought to cause us to not be willing

to permit experimentation that has questionable gain and high
risk from the standpoint of the patient's posture, which is, you
see, the formula that I mentioned we hashed out in our Human Use
Committee."

Involuntarily confined mental patients live in an inherently coercive
institutional environment. Indirect and subtle psychological coercion has
profound effect upon the patient population. Involuntarily confined
patients cannot reason as equals with the doctors and administrators over
whether they should undergo psychosurgery. They are not able to voluntarily give informed consent because of the inherent inequality in their
position.[23]

It has been argued by defendants that because 13 criminal sexual
psychopaths in the Ionia State Hospital wrote a letter indicating they did
not want to be subjects of psychosurgery, that consent can be obtained and
that the arguments about coercive pressure are not valid.

The Court does not feel that this necessarily follows. There is
no showing of the circumstances under which the refusal of these thirteen patients was obtained, and there is no showing whatever that any
effort was made to obtain the consent of these patients for such experimentation.

The fact that thirteen patients unilaterally wrote a letter saying
they did not want to be subjects of psychosurgery is irrelevant to the
question of whether they can consent to that which they are legally precluded from doing.

The law has always been meticulous in scrutinizing inequality in bar-
gaining power and the possibility of undue influence in commercial fields
and in the law of wills. It also has been most careful in excluding from
criminal cases confessions where there was no clear showing of their com-

---

[23]It should be emphasized that once John Doe was released in this case
and returned to the community he withdrew all consent to the performance
of the proposed experiment. His withdrawal of consent under these circumstances should be compared with his response on January 12, 1973, to
questions placed to him by Prof. Slovenko, one of the members of the Human
Rights Committee. These answers are part of exhibit 22 and were given
after extensive publicity about this case, and while John Doe was in
Lafayette Clinic waiting the implantation of depth electrodes. The significant questions and answers are as follows:

1. Would you seek psychosurgery if you were not confined in
    an institution?

A. Yes, if after testing this showed it would be of help.

2. Do you believe that psychosurgery is a way to obtain your
    release from the institution?

A. No, but it would be a step in obtaining my release. It is
    like any other therapy or program to help persons to
    function again.

3. Would you seek psychosurgery if there were other ways to
    obtain your release?

A. Yes. If psychosurgery were the only means of helping my
    physical problem after a period of testing.

pletely voluntary nature after full understanding of the consequences.[24]
No lesser standard can apply to involuntarily detained mental patients.

The keystone to any intrusion upon the body of a person must be full,
adequate and informed consent. The integrity of the individual must be
protected from invasion into his body and personality not voluntarily
agreed to. Consent is not an idle or symbolic act; it is a fundamental
requirement for the protection of the individual's integrity.

We therefore conclude that involuntarily detained mental patients
cannot give informed and adequate consent to experimental psychosurgical
procedures on the brain.

The three basic elements of informed consent--competency, knowledge,
and voluntariness--cannot be ascertained with a degree of reliability
warranting resort to use of such an invasive procedure.[25]

To this point, the Court's central concern has primarily been the
ability of an involuntarily detained mental patient to give a factually
informed, legally adequate consent to psychosurgery. However, there are
also compelling constitutional considerations that preclude the involuntarily detained mental patient from giving effective consent to this type
of surgery.

We deal here with State action in view of the fact the question
relates to involuntarily detained mental patients who are confined because
of the action of the State.

Initially, we consider the application of the First Amendment to the
problem before the Court, recognizing that when the State's interest is in
conflict with the Federal Constitution, the State's interest, even though
declared by statute or court rule, must give way. See NAACP v. Button,
371 U. S. 415 (1963) and United Transportation Workers' Union v. State Bar
of Michigan, 401 U. S. 576 (1971).

A person's mental processes, the communication of ideas, and the
generation of ideas, come within the ambit of the First Amendment. To the

---

[24]See, for example, Miranda v. Arizona, 384 U. S. 436 (1966) and
Escobedo v. Illinois, 378 U. S. 478 (1964).

Prof. Paul Freund of the Harvard Law School has expressed the following opinion:

"I suggest . . . that [prison] experiments should not
involve any promise of parole or of commutation of sentence;
this would be what is called in the law of confessions undue
influence or duress through promise of reward, which can be
as effective in overbearing the will as threats of harm. Nor
should there be a pressure to conform within the prison
generated by the pattern of rejecting parole applications of
those who do not participate. . . ." P. A. Freund, "Ethical
Problems in Human Experimentation," New England Journal of
Medicine, Volume 273 (1965) pages 687-92.

[25]It should be noted that Dr. Vernon H. Mark, a leading psychosurgeon, states that psychosurgery should not be performed on prisoners
who are epileptic because of the problem of obtaining adequate consent.
He states in "Brain Surgery in Aggressive Epileptics," the Hastings
Center Report, Vol. 3, No. 1 (February, 1973): "Prison inmates suffering
from epilepsy should receive only medical treatment; surgical therapy
should not be carried out because of the difficulty in obtaining truly
informed consent."

extent that the First Amendment protects the dissemination of ideas and the expression of thoughts, it equally must protect the individual's right to generate ideas.

As Justice Cardozo pointed out:

"We are free only if we know, and so in proportion to our knowledge. There is no freedom without choice, and there is no choice without knowledge,--or none that is illusory. Implicit, therefore, in the very notion of liberty is the liberty of the mind to absorb and to beget. . . . The mind is in chains when it is without the opportunity to choose. One may argue, if one please, that opportunity to choice is more an evil than a good. One is guilty of a contradiction if one says that the opportunity can be denied, and liberty subsist. At the root of all liberty is the liberty to know. . . .

"Experimentation there may be in many things of deep concern, but not in setting boundaries to thought, for thought freely communicated is the indispensable condition of intelligent experimentation, the one test of its validity.

Cardozo, The Paradoxes of Legal Science, Columbia University Lectures, reprinted in Selected Writings of Benjamin Nathan Cardozo." (Fallon Publications (1947)), pages 317 and 318.

Justice Holmes expressed the basic theory of the First Amendment in Abrams v. United States, 250 U. S. 616, 630 (1919), when he said:

". . . The ultimate good desired is better reached by free trade in ideas--that the best test of truth is the power of the thought to get itself accepted in the competition of the market, and that truth is the only ground upon which their wishes safely can be carried out. That at any rate is the theory of our Constitution. . . . We should be eternally vigilant against attempts to check expressions of opinions that we loathe and believe to be fraught with death, unless they so imminently threaten immediate interference with the lawful and pressing purposes of the law that an immediate check is required to save the country. . . ."

Justice Brandeis in Whitney v. Cal., 274 U. S. 357, 375 (1927), put it this way:

"Those who won our independence believed that the final end of the State was to make men free to value their faculties; and that in its government the deliberative force should prevail over the arbitrary. . . . They believed that freedom to think as you will and to speak as you think are means indispensable to the discovery and spread of political truth; that without free speech and assembly discussion would be futile; that with them, discussion affords ordinarily adequate protection against the dissemination of noxious doctrine; that the greatest menace to freedom is an inert people; that public discussion is a political duty; and that this should be a fundamental principle of the American government. . . ."

Thomas Emerson, a distinguished writer on the First Amendment, stated this in "Toward a General Theory of the First Amendment," 72 Yale Law Journal 877, 895 (1963):

APPENDIX

"The function of the legal process is not only to provide a means whereby a society shapes and controls the behavior of its individual members in the interests of the whole. It also supplies one of the principal methods by which a society controls itself, limiting its own powers in the interests of the individual. The role of the law here is to mark the guide and line between the sphere of social power, organized in the form of the state, and the area of private right. The legal problems involved in maintaining a system of free expression fall largely into this realm. In essence, legal support for such a society involves the protection of individual rights against interference or unwarranted control by the government. More specifically, the legal structure must provide:

"1. Protection of the individual's right to freedom of expression against interference by the government in its efforts to achieve other social objectives or to advance its own interests. . . ."

"3. Restriction of the government in so far as the government itself participates in the system of expression."

"All these requirements involve control over the state. The use of law to achieve this kind of control has been one of the central concerns of freedom-seeking societies over the ages. Legal recognition of individual rights, enforced through the legal processes, has become the core of free society."

In Stanley v. Georgia, 397 U. S. 557 (1969), the Supreme Court once again addressed the free dissemination of ideas. It said at page 565-66:

"Our whole constitutional heritage rebels at the thought of giving government the power to control men's minds. . . . Whatever the power of the state to control dissemination of ideas inimical to public morality, it cannot constitutionally premise legislation on the desirability of controlling a person's private thoughts."

Freedom of speech and expression, and the right of all men to disseminate ideas, popular or unpopular, are fundamental to ordered liberty. Government has no power or right to control men's minds, thoughts, and expressions. This is the command of the First Amendment. And we adhere to it in holding an involuntarily detained mental patient may not consent to experimental psychosurgery.

For, if the First Amendment protects the freedom to express ideas, it necessarily follows that it must protect the freedom to generate ideas. Without the latter protection, the former is meaningless.

Experimental psychosurgery, which is irreversible and intrusive, often leads to the blunting of emotions, the deadening of memory, the reduction of affect, and limits the ability to generate new ideas. Its potential for injury to the creativity of the individual is great, and can impinge upon the right of the individual to be free from interference with his mental processes.

The State's interest in performing psychosurgery and the legal ability of the involuntarily detained mental patient to give consent must bow to the First Amendment, which protects the generation and free flow of ideas from unwarranted interference with one's mental processes.

To allow an involuntarily detained mental patient to consent to the type of psychosurgery proposed in this case, and to permit the State to perform it, would be to condone State action in violation of basic First Amendment rights of such patients, because impairing the power to generate ideas inhibits the full dissemination of ideas.

There is no showing in this case that the State has met its burden of demonstrating such a compelling State interest in the use of experimental psychosurgery on involuntarily detained mental patients to overcome its proscription by the First Amendment of the United States Constitution.

In recent years, the Supreme Court of the United States has developed a constitutional concept of right of privacy, relying upon the First, Fifth and Fourteenth Amendments. It was found in the marital bed in Griswold v. Conn., 381 U. S. 479 (1962); in the right to view obscenity in the privacy of one's home in Stanley v. Georgia, 395 U. S. 557 (1969); and in the right of a woman to control her own body by determining whether she wishes to terminate a pregnancy in Rowe v. Wade, 41 L W 4213 (1973).

The concept was also recognized in the case of a prison inmate subjected to shock treatment and an experimental drug without his consent in Mackey v. Procunier, _____ F 2d _____, 71-3062 (9th Circuit, April 16, 1973).

In that case, the 9th Circuit noted that the District Court had treated the action as a malpractice claim and had dismissed it. The 9th Circuit reversed, saying, inter alia:

> "It is asserted in memoranda that the staff at Vacaville is engaged in medical and psychiatric experimentation with 'aversion treatment' of criminal offenders, including the use of succinycholine on fully conscious patients. It is emphasized the plaintiff was subject to experimentation without consent.

> "Proof of such matters could, in our judgment, raise serious constitutional questions respecting cruel and unusual punishment or impermissable tinkering with the mental processes. (Citing Stanley among other cases.) In our judgment it was error to dismiss the case without ascertaining at least the extent to which such charges can be substantiated. . . ." (Emphasis added).

Much of the rationale for the developing constitutional concept of right to privacy is found in Justice Brandeis' famous dissent in Olmstead v. United States, 277 U. S. 438 (1928), at 478, where he said:

> "The makers of our Constitution undertook to secure conditions favorable to the pursuit of happiness. They recognized the significance of man's spiritual nature, of his feelings and of his intellect. They knew that only a part of the pain, pleasure, and satisfaction of life are to be found in material things. They sought to protect Americans in their beliefs, their thoughts, their emotions and their sensations. They conferred, as against the Government, the right to be let alone--the most comprehensive of rights and the right most valued by civilized men."

There is no privacy more deserving of constitutional protection than that of one's mind. As pointed out by the Court in Huguez v. United States, 406 F 2d 366 (1968), at page 382, footnote 84:

> ". . . Nor are the intimate internal areas of the physical habitation of mind and soul any less deserving of precious preservation from unwarranted and forcible intrusions than are the intimate internal areas of the physical habitation of wife and family. Is not the sanctity of the body even more important, and

therefore, more to be honored in its protection than the sanc-
tity of the home? . . ."

Intrusion into one's intellect, when one is involuntarily detained and
subject to the control of institutional authorities, is an intrusion into
one's constitutionally protected right of privacy. If one is not protected
in his thoughts, behavior, personality and identity, then the right of
privacy becomes meaningless.[26]

Before a State can violate one's constitutionally protected right of
privacy and obtain a valid consent for experimental psychosurgery on
involuntarily detained mental patients, a compelling State interest must
be shown. None has been shown here.

To hold that the right of privacy prevents laws against dissemination
of contraceptive material as in <u>Griswold</u> v. <u>Conn</u>. (supra), or the right to
view obscenity in the privacy of one's home as in <u>Stanley</u> v. <u>Georgia</u>
(supra), but that it does not extend to the physical intrusion in an
experimental manner upon the brain of an involuntarily detained mental
patient is to denigrate the right. In the hierarchy of values, it is more
important to protect one's mental processes than to protect even the
privacy of the marital bed. To authorize an involuntarily detained mental
patient to consent to experimental psychosurgery would be to fail to
recognize and follow the mandates of the Supreme Court of the United
States, which has constitutionally protected the privacy of body and mind.

Counsel for John Doe has argued persuasively that the use of the
psychosurgery proposed in the instant case would constitute cruel and
unusual punishment and should be barred under the Eighth Amendment. A
determination of this issue is not necessary to decision, because of the
many other legal and constitutional reasons for holding that the involuntarily detained mental patient may not give an informed and valid consent
to experimental psychosurgery. We therefore do not pass on the issue of
whether the psychosurgery proposed in this case constitutes cruel and
unusual punishment within the meaning of the Eighth Amendment.

For the reasons given, we conclude that the answer to question number
one posed for decision is no.

In reaching this conclusion, we emphasize two things.

First, the conclusion is based upon the state of the knowledge as of
the time of the writing of this Opinion. When the state of medical knowledge develops to the extent that the type of psychosurgical intervention
proposed here becomes an accepted neurosurgical procedure and is no longer
experimental, it is possible, with appropriate review mechanisms,[27] that
involuntarily detained mental patients could consent to such an operation.

Second, we specifically hold that an involuntarily detained mental
patient today can give adequate consent to accepted neurosurgical procedures.

In view of the fact we have answered the first question in the negative, it is not necessary to proceed to a consideration of the second
question, although we cannot refrain from noting that had the answer to
the first question been yes, serious constitutional problems would have
arisen with reference to the second question.

---

[26]See Note: 45 <u>So. Cal. L R</u> 616, 663 (1972).

[27]For example, see Guidelines of the Department of Health, Education
and Welfare, A C Exhibit 17.

One final word. The Court thanks all counsel for the excellent, lawyer-like manner in which they have conducted themselves. Seldom, if ever, has any member of this panel presided over a case where the lawyers were so well-prepared and so helpful to the Court.

The findings in this Opinion shall constitute the findings of fact and conclusions of law upon the issues framed pursuant to the provisions of G.C.R. (1963) 517.1.

A judgment embodying the findings of the Court in this Opinion may be presented.

HORACE W. GILMORE
Circuit Judge

GEORGE E. BOWLES
Circuit Judge

JOHN D. O'HAIR
Circuit Judge

Detroit, Michigan

July 10, 1973

APPENDIX

GABE KAIMOWITZ, representing himself and certain individual members of the Medical Committee for Human Rights on behalf of JOHN DOE and at least 23 others similarly situated who are held or committed involuntarily in public institutions in Michigan,
 	
                Petitioner - Plaintiffs,
 	
-VS-
 	
DEPARTMENT OF MENTAL HEALTH FOR THE STATE OF MICHIGAN, DR. E. G. YUDASHKIN, Director, State Department of Mental Health; DR. J. S. GOTTLIEB, Director, Lafayette Clinic; DR. ERNST RODIN, Associate of Dr. Gottlieb at the Clinic, in their official capacities, as well as their agents, assignees, employees, and successors in office,
 	
                Respondents - Defendants.
	))	CIVIL ACTION NO. 73-19434-AW

A P P E N D I X

ITEM NO. 1.   PROPOSAL FOR THE STUDY OF THE TREATMENT OF
UNCONTROLLABLE AGGRESSION AT THE LAFAYETTE CLINIC,
by J. S. Gottlieb, M. D. and Ernst A. Rodin, M. D.,
Exhibit A.

It is proposed that a study be carried out to investigate the results of medical versus surgical treatment of patients who have been committed to the state hospital system because of severe uncontrollable aggressive outbursts. Within the state hospital system, particularly at Ionia, there exist patients who must be continually hospitalized for many years because of uncontrollable aggressive behavior with or without sexual connotations. It has been shown that spontaneous uncontrolled aggressive behavior is accompanied, in certain individuals, by marked electrical abnormalities in portions of the brain: the limbic system, especially: amygdaloid nucleus, fornix, and cingulate gyrus. It has also been shown that these behavioral outbursts can be triggered by remote stimulation of the brain through implanted electrodes. It has been claimed that when the area which triggers these discharges is destroyed by cauterization or surgical removal, the patient will no longer suffer from these disturbances. It has also been claimed that it is possible to restore certain patients to a useful life in the community through these operative interventions. It is therefore suggested that the Lafayette Clinic conduct a controlled study on the value of these operative procedures in the hope that some patients, who are now permanently institutionalized, can be restored to the community.

Patients who are now in the state hospital system, especially Ionia, and whose relatives as well as the patient himself would be willing to have brain surgery performed would be transferred to the Lafayette Clinic.

206

After initial neurological, psychiatric and psychological evaluations, depth electrodes would be implanted by Dr. Ortiz at Providence Hospital or members of the department of neurosurgery of Wayne State University at Grace Hospital, into strategic locations of the patient's brain. This procedure takes about one-half day and the patient would then be returned to Lafayette Clinic for continued study over a period of approximately one month. During this time, extensive electroencephalographic work-up of the patient would be accomplished in the laboratory setting, as well as on the ward where the patient's interactions with ward personnel and other patients can be monitored and manipulated. The depthelectrogram would be monitored by telemetry, and electrical stimulation of various discrete brain structures carried out under different amounts of environment stress. After an area of abnormal function has been identified by conventional means, as well as computer analysis of the data, the patient will be returned to Providence or Grace Hospital for removal of electrodes and definitive surgery to eliminate that particular structure. If the offending area is quite small, electro-coagulation will be done; if the area is quite large, block resection will be performed. The removed tissue will be subjected to histological and histochemical analysis for the possible detection of specific abnormalities. After the immediate postoperative recovery period, estimated at about five days, the patient will be returned to the Lafayette Clinic where extensive psychological testing will be repeated to determine whether or not specific postoperative deficits in cognitive or emotional functions can be detected, and whether or not improvement in certain areas of behavior can be objectively demonstrated.

With the help of a social worker and a rehabilitation counselor, a maximum effort will then be made to place the patient in the community into an environment that will allow him to live up to his potential. If a patient were to show after depth implantation no significant electrographic abnormalities, the electrodes will be withdrawn without the setting of a lesion. The evaluation of the patient during the time he has electrodes implanted will take about one month and one can therefore study and treat approximately 12 patients in this manner during a one year period.

To guard against operating on patients in whom the medical indication might be dubious, a Committee was formed which will review the abstracted charts of all patients referred by the state hospitals. The Committee consists of Dr. Murray Thomas--Chairman of the Department of Neurosurgery at Wayne State University; Dr. John Gilroy--Chairman of the Department of Neurology at Wayne State University; and Dr. Elliot Luby of the Lafayette Clinic.

To guard against infringement of the human rights of the patients who have been selected by the mentioned physicians another committee was formed. This committee consists of a representative of the clergy--Monsignor Clifford Sawher; the legal profession--Professor Slovenko of Wayne State University; and a community representative--Mr. Frank Moran of Southfield. This committee reviews the Informed Consent form and may wish to interview the prospective patient prior to his transfer to the Lafayette Clinic. After a patient has been cleared by the Medical Committee, the procedure will be explained to him and his family by a member of the Department of Neurology of Lafayette Clinic while he is still residing at his state hospital. The patient and the family will also be given the Informed Consent sheet, these will be left with them for at least a week during which time they have the opportunity to weigh the pros and cons of the suggested procedure.

As a corollary to this study, it is proposed that we evaluate also a purely medical approach to the problem based on the fact that the hormone responsible for aggressive behavior is, in all probability, testosterone. An antiandrogen substance has recently been synthesized and has been used in Europe in the treatment of severe sexual psychopathy with associated aggressive behavior. It is therefore proposed that as a control group, 10 to 12 patients from the state hospital system who are matched for sex, age, intellectual level and similarity of episodic behavioral disturbances be transferred on an individual basis to the Lafayette Clinic and, after initial work-up, their testicular function will be depressed by anti-androgens. Environmental manipulation and psychological evaluations will be similar to that which is being carried out in the surgical candidates and serum androgen levels will be monitored. If it can be shown that the antiandrogens do indeed induce a marked calming effect and increase the stress tolerance to a degree that the patient is safe for life in the com-munity, he will likewise receive maximum benefit of rehabilitative services. The successful cases will be placed on convalescent status and followed closely by the Lafayette Clinic; unsuccessful patients will be returned to Ionia State Hospital. The best antiandrogen is cyproterone acetate produced by the Schering Corporation in West Germany. It is not available at this time in the United States although negotiations have been started between the Schering Corporation and Lafayette Clinic to provide us with some of the material for experimental use.

If the surgical group proves to have a superior success rate, the medically treated group could then be worked-up surgically at a later date. If, on the other hand, medical treatment could be proven to be just as effective as surgery, it would allow the treatment of a much larger patient population in the future because of its basic simplicity.

The project has already been funded for the current fiscal year by the State Legislature.

ITEM NO. 2.   CRITERIA FOR INCLUSION IN AGGRESSION PROJECT,
              Amicus Curiae Exhibit 2

Since the purpose of the project is to render habitually aggressive patients safe for living in the community, the following guidelines for patient selection have been drawn up.

1) Patient's age 25 or over.

2) Sex should be male in the first 6 to 7 patients.

3) Patient should have been in the State Mental Hospital System because of predominantly aggressive behavior for at least 5 years and should be regarded as being treatment resistant to conventional methods.

4) The Full Scale I. Q. should be at least 80.

5) The patient should not suffer from paranoid ideation.

6) The patient should not suffer from a schizophrenic psychosis even if it does not contain paranoid features.

7) The patient should have had several attacks of severe aggressive behavior with or without the use of alcohol and with or without sexual connotations.

8) The patient should remember his acts of violence and experience a certain amount of remorse while claiming that he was unable to prevent himself from committing the aggressive actions.

9) The patient should be mentally competent to the extent that he fully comprehends the procedure of depthelectrography and possible stereo-tactic surgery. He must be able to give his voluntary informed consent.

10) Voluntary Informed Consent must also be obtained from the responsible relatives or guardians.

REASONS FOR THE STIPULATIONS:

Ad 1) Age of 25 is minimal to assess chronicity of disorder and will act as a preventive measure that operation might be performed on patients who could benefit from continued conventional medical treatment.

2) It has been shown that unprovoked acts of aggression are carried out mostly by males; if females are severely aggressive they tend to have diffuse brain disease which could not be expected to yield to focal elimination of a given brain structure.

3) This point gives further evidence for the chronicity of the patient's illness and his poor prognosis without drastic intervention.

4) Patients with I. Q.'s below 80 are not likely to become self-sustaining citizens in our complex society even if the symptom of aggression were to be removed.

5) Patients with paranoid ideation will continue to remain incapacitated because of their paranoia and will, furthermore, incorporate any attempt at therapy utilizing depth-electrodes into their delusional system making them thereby potentially even more dangerous.

6) The schizophrenic psychosis will remain uninfluenced by stereotactic surgery and the patient will be in need of continued hospitalization.

7) Since an isolated act of violence including rape or murder may not recur in a patient's lifetime, only those patients should be investigated who have a high recurrence risk.

8) 9)
& 10) Ensure a genuine interest on part of the patient and his family to explore the help that might be derived from experimental treatment approaches.

INDEX

Abrams v. *United States*, 201
affective psychosis, 65
aggressive behavior, *see* violent behavior
Albert Einstein College of Medicine, *VIII*
American Medical Association, Guidelines on Clinical Investigation, 125, 127
American Orthopsychiatric Association, 74-75, 188
amygdala: amygdalotomy, 47, 48, 49, 50, 56, 80; experimental lesions and, 39; as part of limbic system, 37, 54; stereotacic lesioning of, 47; violent behavior and, 49, 56
angina, 14
antibiotics, 15
antisepsis, 15
anxiety, 17; reduction of, postlobotomy, 42; reduction of, via ESB, 63
automatons, 4, 19
autonomic nervous system, 35-36, 38
avoidance, active and passive, 31

Balasubramanian, V., 192
Bard, P., 37
Bartholow, Roberts, 55
Beall, Sen. J. Glenn, 10
behavior control: books and movies on, 205; defining "optimal" behavior, 61; ethical problems of, 88; genetics and, 118; motive for psychosurgery, 119-20; new forms of, 4; personal identity and, 93-94, 96; potential for misuse, 5-6; psychosurgery definition and, 118; reinforcement and, 60, 61-62; reward and punishment, 4, 57, 60; self-regulated, 57, 61, 63; social systems of, 3; success of science and, 4;
Beyond Freedom and Dignity (Skinner), 22
Bianchi, L., 32, 33
biofeedback, 61
biological psychiatry, 25, 26
Boston Psychopathic Hospital, 41
Bowles, Judge George E., 188, 192n.
brain; cognitive function potential, 34; complexity of, 37, 177; dichotomy of mind and, 29, 46; environment and, 89-96, 116, 177; ethical problems concerning PMB and, 88; frontal lobe functions, 35-36; functional recovery of, following lesions, 38, 39, 53, 162; integration of systems, 38-39; mapping of cortex, 55-56; reversible depression of function, 45; self-manipulation of, 61; temporal lobe functions, 36; *see also* limbic system
brainwashing, 19
Brandeis, Justice Louis D., 201
Breggin, Peter, 10, 16, 124, 190
Brown, Bertram S., 119, 120, 189, 190
Bucy, P. C., 32, 33
Burt, Prof. Robert A., 188

California Organic Therapy Law, 157
cannula, 119
Cardozo, Justice Benjamin N., 201
chemical stimulation of the brain, 6, 45; operating mechanisms of, 28; potential for misuse, 28; selectivity of, 58; therapeutic potential of, 59-60
cingulate gyri, 37
Columbia College of Physicians and Surgeons, *VIII*
Columbia-Greystone Associates, 35, 41
Columbia University School of Law, *IX*
Congressional Record, 10
Congress of Neurology (1935), 40
consent (to psychosurgery), 12-13, 138-160, 320-27; allowance of, 138-45; ascertaining appropriate, 145-49; by the competent adult, 138-49; criminal rehabilitation and, 160-64, 183; drug experimentation and, 133; "informed," 12, 108-13, 123, 126, 130; irreversibility of psychosurgery and, 142-44; medical model and, 145-46, 151; medical opinions and, 139, 141-42, 146-47; medical problems and, 139-42; moratorium on patients unable to give full, 152; potential for abuse of, 154-55, 160-61; proxy, 13-14, 138, 149-60, 189;

questions concerning, 87-88, 92-93; side-effects and, 145; under influence of drugs, 158
control groups, 9
Cooper, I., 127
cost-benefit analysis, *VII*
culture and man, 3, 20

Delgado, Jose M. R., 57, 80, 141
depression, 17; as intrapersonal disease, 18; reduction of, postlobotomy, 42
depth psychology, 4
Descartes, René, 29
Detroit Free Press, 74, 84, 187
Detroit psychosurgery case, *see* *Kaimowitz* v. *Department of Mental Health of the State of Michigan*
drugs: antipsychotic, 43, 54; chemical stimulation of the brain, 58; chloropromazine, 137; contrast of surgery and, 133-36; "curing" personality disorders, 53; failure of, 26; FDA and, 123, 128-29, 133-36, 149; influence of, and consent, 158; irreversibility of effects, 26; mass delivery methods, 5; narcotics, 64; "new drugs," 133-34; as organic therapy, 17; "performance" type, 142; reversibility of effects, 24; specialized nature of, 4; surgical contract and, 7; testosterone, 77; thalidomide, 149; therapeutic value of, 14-15, 44; thorazine, 159; totalitarian control and, 19, 137, 179; tranquilizers, 8, 17, 170; Urokon, 135
Duke University, *VIII*
duodenum, 16-17
dycrasias, blood, 17
dystonia, 45, 127

"ecology movement," 5
Edgar, Harold, *IX*, 7, 117-68
electrical stimulation of the brain (ESB), 54-63; behavioral and physiological effect of, 57, 58; characteristics of, 27; cortical response to, 55; environmental manipulation and, 60, 61-62; epilepsy as natural counterpart of, 54; first modification of behavior by, 55; inducing violence and, 56; lasting

changes in mood via, 62; as negative reinforcement, 57; operating mechanisms of, 28; as positive reinforcement, 27; potential for misuse of, 28; remote control devices and, 4; self stimulation phenomenon, 57; therapeutic potential of, 59-60
electrode implantation, 6; depthelectrodes, 73, 80; idea implanting and, 21; as means of political control, 19; via stereotacic techniques, 60
electroencephalography: epilepsy and, 17, 46; Kaimowitz case and, 78, 82; violence and, 49
Emerson, Thomas, 201-202
endocrine glands, 38
epilepsy: amygdalotomy and, 50; artificial induction of seizures, 55; as behavior disturbance, 25; as clue to brain functioning, 29; definition of, 54; EEG and, 17, 46; ESB potential and, 28, 59; frontal lobe, 16; functional neurosurgery and, 45; seizures, 36, 54, 172, 173; surgical treatment of, 46-47; temporal lobe, 16, 18, 36, 49, 80; violence and, 16, 49, 120, 160, 173; *Violence and the Brain* and, 80, 124
equipotentiality, 34
Ervin, Frank, 75-77, 190, 190n., 191, 191n.; amygdalotomy and violence, 48-49; epilepsy and violence, 15-16; mood changes via ESB, 62; psychosurgery and rioters, 160
"experimental neurosis," 40
experimentation: AMA's Guidelines on Clinical Investigation, 125, 220; animal model limitations, 27, 30-31, 32, 36, 57; "critical" sites for lobotomy, 44; definition of, 14; drugs and, 133-34; early, 30; effects of brain lesions on behavior, 29-39; with ESB, 56-57; ethics and, 125-29; functional map of human cortex and, 56; lobectomy, 32-33; lobotomy in monkeys, 40; malpractice and, 229-31; mechanisms for safeguarding, 27, 66-67, 118; need for in PMB, 67-70; in PMB techniques, 28; as status of psychosurgery, 176-78; with stereotacic methods, 45; of therapeutic brain stimulation, 60-61; trial and error of biological therapies, 25
Experimentation with Human Beings (Katz), 194

Falconer (British neurosurgeon), 49
First Amendment, 200-204, 264-65
Flourens, Pierre, 33-34
Foerster, Otfrid, 55-56
Food and Drug Administration (FDA),
    123, 128-29, 133-36, 149, 167n.
Freeman, Walter, 8, 40, 42
Freund, Prof. P. A., 200n.
Fritsch, G., 55
Fulton, J. F., 40
functional neurosurgery, 45

Gallagher, Rep. Cornelius, 10
Gass, Ronald S., *VIII*, 73-86
Gaylin, William M., *VII-VIII*, 3-23
George Washington University Medical
    School, 8
Gilroy, Judge John, 207
Gottlieb, J. S., 73, 76-77, 80, 81, 186,
    187, 190n., 194, 206-209
Griswold v. Connecticut, 203, 204

Hastings Institute Conference on Physi-
    cal Brain Manipulation, 141
Health, Education and Welfare, Depart-
    ment of (HEW), 123
Heath, Robert: environmental manipula-
    tion and ESB, 60; mood changes via
    ESB, 62; self-stimulation in schizo-
    phrenia, 57
Hess, W. R., 56
hippocampus: memory loss and, 47; as
    part of limbic system, 37, 54; process
    of learning and, 36-37
Hippocrates, 29, 64
Hitzig, E., 55
homosexuality, 60, 99
Holmes, Justice Oliver Wendell, 201
Horsley, Sir Victor, 55
Hortner v. Koch, 195
Huguez v. United States, 203-204
hypersexuality: amygdala lesions and,
    39; criminal behavior and, 52, 53;
    Kaimowitz case and, 77, 79; limbic
    system and, 38; sex hormones and, 38
hypothalamus: aphagia and, 39; ESB and,
    57; hypothalamotomy, 48, 56; integra-
    tion of, with brain systems, 38; loca-
    tion of, 36; as part of limbic system,

37; violent behavior and, 37, 49,
    53, 56

infarction, 14
Institute of Society, Ethics and the Life
    Sciences, *VII, VIII, IX*, 6; Behavioral
    Control Research Group of, *VII, IX*, 6
Ionia State Hospital, 79, 80, 82, 185, 186,
    198, 199, 206, 208

Jackson, J. Hughlings, 54-55
Jacobsen, C. F., 35, 40
*Kaimowitz v. Department of Mental Health
    of the State of Michigan,* 73-85, 124-25,
    152-43, 155, 185-209; consent and
    review procedures, 82, 193-200; court
    opinion, 152-153, 312-14; "criteria for
    inclusion in aggression project," 78-79;
    design of study, 73, 206-209; EEG
    difficulties, 78; Human and Animal
    Experimentation Committee, 80-81,
    82-83; investigation by Gabe Kaimo-
    witz, 84; John Doe and, 79-84, 185-87;
    Michigan legislature and, 78; Michigan
    Medical Committee for Human Rights,
    74; preparations for electrode implan-
    tation, 83; prologue to court opinion,
    75-84; proxy consent and, 153, 189;
    questions for declaratory judgment, 75;
    review committees, 81, 83, 187, 207;
    revision of criteria, 80; termination of
    project funding, 84; testosterone and,
    77; unresolved legal dilemmas, 84-85;
    Violence and the Brain and, 75-77
Kalamazoo County Circuit Court, 185
Katz, Jay, 194
Klüver, H., 32, 33
Klüver-Bucy syndrome, 36

Lafayette Clinic, 73-85 *passim*, 185-209
    passim
lasers, 119
Lashley, Karl, 33-34
lesions: adaptability and, 35; of the
    amygdala, 39; assault upon the soul
    and, 46; as basis for frontal lobotomy,
    35; behavior alterations and, 31, 32;

cognitive functions and, 34; complex effects of, 32, 33; deep within the brain, 37; of drive related brain regions, 53; evaluation of new sites, 45; functional neurosurgery and, 45-46; function recovery of brain following, 38, 39, 53, 162; inferior and medial frontal lobe, 44; of limbic system, 38; localizationist theory and, 34; motor and sensory deficits caused by, 33; of orbital and medial cortex, 36; space-occupying, 16; stereotacic production of, 45

Lima, Almeida, 40

limbic system: composition of, 37-38; criminal behavior and, 51-52; definition of, 8; ESB behavior modifications and, 57, 60, 62; as focal point of epileptic seizures, 54-55; monitoring of, by depthelectrodes, 73; prefrontal lobotomy and, 8; region of, 36; violent behavior and, 38, 48-49; *see also* amygdala

lithium, 18

lobectomy, 32-33, 47

lobotomy, frontal, 192n.; antipsychotic drugs and, 43; current surgical approaches to, 36; empirical basis for, 35; first performed, 39-40; frequency of operations, 40, 43; "frontal lobe syndrome," 42; intellectual deterioration following, 41; intractable pain and, 50; memory loss and, 47; nonexistance of follow up studies, 42, 43; regional variations in method, 41; seeking specificity of results, 43; therapeutic effects of, 42, 53; transorbital technique, 40-41; use of, in institutions, 48, 160

lobotomy, prefrontal, 160; abuse of, 8-9; modern procedures, 8, 14; numbers of, performed, 9; as original psychosurgery, 7-8; supplanted by drugs, 8

localization, 34

London, Perry, 94

Luby, Elliot, 187, 207

"machine model of man," 94

Mackey v. *Propcunier*, 168n., 205, 295n.

manic-depressive psychosis, 18

Mark, Vernon, 75-77, 200n.; amygdalot-

omy and violence, 48-49; epilepsy and violence, 15-16; Kaimowitz case and, 80, 190, 190n., 191, 191n.; mood changes via ESB, 62; organic criteria of psychosurgery, 16; psychosurgery and rioters, 160

mass media: access to means of, 5; con-control through, 6, 19, 308; indoctrination and, 5

Meister, Joel S., *IX*, 7, 169-84

mental illness: assessment of therapy, 44-45; biochemical abnormalities underlying, 58-59; complex origins of, 25; defining of, 63, 118, 172-73; diagnosis of, 64-65, 66-67; first attempt to ameliorate, via surgery, 39-40; individual quality of, 9; "informed" consent and, 13; national distinctions in diagnosis, 65; NIMH grant, 15n.; severity of, and psychosurgery, 24; stigma of, 20; *see also* schizophrenia

mental institutions: "appropriate" treatment in, 159; chloropromazine at, 137; custodial use of therapeutic devices, 19; dependency of life within, 153; in Japan, 48; population reductions in, 43; proxy consent and, 149-150; Russian exploitation of, 20; thorazine at, 159

Michels, Robert, 120

Miller, N. E., 57

Milner, Brenda, 36, 47

mind, 29, 46

minimal brain dysfunction, 170

Model Penal Code, 144

Moniz, Egas, 40

Montreal Neurological Institute, 56

Moran, Frank, 187, 207

Narabayashi (Japanese neurosurgeon), 47, 48

National Commission for the Protection of Human Subjects of Biomedical and Behavioral Research, 181

National Institute of Mental Health (NIMH): clinical evaluation of psychiatric disorders and, 43; conference on Psychosurgery, 69; grant, 15n., statistics compiled by, 41

Neuro-Research Foundation, Boston, 15n.

Neville, Robert, *IX*, 87-116

New York Mental Hygiene Law, 159
"normalcy": culture and, 151-52, 156-58; difficulty in defining, 20, 63, 88, 97-99; health and, 100-104, 116; medical coercion and, 21
Nuremberg Code, 67, 195-97, 198

obligatory external controls, 3
O'Hair, Judge John D., 188
Olmstead v. *United States*, 203

pain: in animal experimentation, 31; frontal lobotomy and, 50; functional neurosurgery and, 45, 46; reduction of, via ESB, 63, 121, 173, 174
Parkinsonism: "behavior" control and, 120; functional neurosurgery and, 45; L. dopa and, 129; as organic condition, 46; stereotacic surgery and, 47
peer pressure, 3
Penfield, Wilder, 46, 56
peptic ulcer, 16-17
Physical Control of the Mind (Delgado), 111
physical manipulation of the brain (PMB), 6, 63-70; "art" of medicine and, 64; biological therapies and, 66; need for experimentation, 67-70; special status of, 24; *see also* chemical stimulation of the brain; electrical stimulation of the brain; psychosurgery
psychosurgery: conditions warranting, 174-76; contemporary, 43-47; controversy surrounding, 9-11, 47, 48, 54; definition of, 7, 24, 119-20, 172-76; delivery system for, 150; dramatic nature of, 6, 7, 178; effects of brain lesions on behavior, 29-39; effects of treatment criteria for, 175-76; environmental manipulation and, 61; evaluation of, 27, 37, 39, 44, 61, 68-69, 177-78; experimental status of, 176-78; experimental versus therapeutic, 13-15, 176; functional recovery of brain following, 38, 39, 53, 162; fundamental concern of, 25, 94; human autonomy and, 21-22; implications of, 4-5; irreversibility of, 9, 21, 27, 54, 119, 142-44, 178; Kaimowitz case,

73-85, 312-36; medical contract and, 19-20; "mentalistic" definition of, 51; motives criteria for, 119-20, 172-74, 175, 183; "normalcy" and, 20; organic versus nonorganic, 15-18, 46, 50-51, 52, 66-67, 142-45, 163, 174; original, 7-8, 9; potential for misuse, 6, 10; as prototype of behavior modification, 6-7; as "psychiatric neurosurgery," 172; regulating, 180-83; religious influence and, 5; restricted use of, 24; as "surgery of violence," 171; surgical contract and, 7; therapeutic context of, 24; therapy versus social control, 18-19, 51, 118, 121, 179; therapy versus social engineering, 19-21; totalitarianism and, 19; understanding brain mechanisms and, 28; unpredictable results of, 27, 54, 177; untoward effects of, 28, 42, 43, 145, 173, 177; as viable alternative to criminal behavior, 117-18; violence and, 47-54; *see also* consent (to psychosurgery)
psychosurgery, ethical and moral aspects of, 11, 59, 87-116; brain as environment for the self, 90-92; coercion factor, 20-21, 110, 144; environment and brain, 89-96; experimentation, 125-29; guaranteed efficiency, 106; human autonomy, 21-22; institutionalization or psychosurgery, 152; internal and external environments, 93-96, 172-73; medical opinions, 138-139, 141-42, 146-47; "normal" to "healthy," 100-104; personal respect, 106, 121-22; questions concerning, 87-89; social control, 104-107, 113-15; social cost, 106-107; therapeutic control, 96-104, 108-13; who controls?, 107-15; *see also* consent (to psychosurgery)
psychosurgery, legal aspects of, 10-11, 15, 117-68; AMA's Guidelines on Clinical investigation, 125, 127; assessment based on acts not intentions, 174; California Organic Therapy Law, 156; control mechanisms, 122-23; criminal behavior, 117; cruel and unusual punishment, 161; data collection, 123-29, 136, 177; drug/surgery contrast, 133-36; federal regulations, 131-32, 133-36; First Amendment, 153-54; group decision making, 128; hospitals and, 131;

imposed treatment, 159-60; Kaimowitz case, 73-85, 185-207; legislation, 136-37, 148-49; locality rule, 129, 135; maiming, 139; malpractice, 122-23, 129-31; medical model, 145-46, 151, 159; motive and, 119-20; New York Mental Hygiene Law, 159-60; Nuremberg Code, 67, 195-97, 198; parole and, 162, 179; patients propensity to sue, 130; penal policy, 161-65, 285n.-286n.; "professions" and, 131, 135, 140; protection of judicial processes, 156-57; "psychosurgery board," 136-137, 148; record keeping, 128; redefining values, 20-21; regulations, 121-39, 195-97; review committees, 132, 147-48; right of refusal, 160; self-regulation of experimentation, 118, 122, 130-32, 148; semantic problems, 120-21; specific criminal behavior intervention, 163-64; stigmatization, 141, 150; Stokes bill, 181-82; terminology, 119-22; "unconscionable" contracts, 156-57; *see also* consent (to psychosurgery)

psychosurgery, political and social aspects of, 10-11, 15, 52, 114-15, 116, 169-81; control of medical innovation, 171; economic base of medical care, 170, 179-80; in Japan, 48, 152; malevolent government, 19, 118, 137-138; Medhvedev case, 20; "myth" of mental illness, 65; nature of disorders, 46; "normalcy," 156-58; penal policy, 162; politicization of medicine, 169-72; rioters and, 160; social abuse, 178-80; social context of, 171; *see also* consent (to psychosurgery)

Psychosurgery: Proceeding of the Second International Conference, 43-44

Radical Therapist, The, 98
Ranson, S. W., 56
remote control electronic devices, 4
Roberts, W. W., 57
Rodin, Ernst, 73-84, 124, 186, 187, 194, 197, 206-209
Rowe v. *Wade*, 203
Russia, 20, 118

Salgo v. *Leland Stanford Jr. University Board of Trust*, 135
Sano (Japanese neurosurgeon), 48
Sawher, Monsignor Clifford, 187, 207
Schering Corporation, 208
schizophrenia: ESB and, 57; lobotomy and, 41-42, 65; national distinctions in diagnosis, 65; psychosurgery and, 4, 177; temporal lobe excisions and, 36
Scoville, W. B., 36, 47
"sedative surgery," 48
self: autonomy, 21-22; brain as environment for, 90-92, 95; destruction of, 25; emotional components of, 13; ethical problems concerning PMB and, 88; intrusion upon, 46, 106, 118, 121, 137, 142; personality change and, 96, 137
self-control, 101-102
Senate Joint Resolution 86, 10
sepsis, 15
septal region, 37
shock treatment, 8
Skinner, B. F., 19, 22, 62
Slovenko, Ralph, 187, 199n., 207
soul: assault upon, 46; as highest part of man, 10; "humanness," 137; as unifying principle of the body, 116
Stanley v. *Georgia*, 202-203, 204
State University of New York at Purchase, IX
stereotaxic devices: amygdalotomy, 47, 50; assault upon the soul and, 46; electrical or chemical stimulation and, 60; electrode implantation and, 60, 73-74, 176; for prefrontal lobotomy, 8; for producing brain lesions, 45
Stokes, Rep. L. H. R., 181
stress: brain lesions and, 34
"style," 102-103
surgery, general, 7, 15, 16, 17, 167n.
Sweet, William H.: psychological deficits postlobotomy, 50; violence and temporal lobe epilepsy, 15-16; violent behavior and brain changes, 18-19

"taste makers," 5
thalamic nuclei, 37, 40
Thomas, Murray, 207
topectomy, 35
tumor, brain, 16, 55, 119

United States v. *Karl Brandt*, 195-97
University of California at Los Angeles
  (UCLA), 10-11

Vaughan, Herbert G., Jr., *VIII*, 7, 24-72
Veatch, Robert, 11
Violence and the Brain (Mark and Ervin),
  18, 48, 75, 76, 80, 83, 124, 191
violent behavior: amygdala and, 39, 49,
  56; brain changes and, 18-19; brain
  pathology and, 26, 52-53; complex
  origins of, 56-57; "curing" personality disorders, 53; as drive related, 38;
  epilepsy and, 16, 49, 120, 160; hypothalamus and, 37, 49, 56; induced by
  ESB, 56; as interpersonal disease, 18,
  117; Kaimowitz case and, 73-85;
  limbic system and, 38; management
  of, 47-48, 52; modification of, via ESB,
  62-63; potential damage of present-
day, 117; psychosurgery and penal
  policy, 160-64, 164n.-165n., 168n.;
  taxic amygdalotomy and, 47, 48;
  study of, 10-11, 15n.; types of, 52
volitional controls, 3

Watson, (doctor), 198-99
Watts, James, 40
West, Louis Jolyon, 10-11
Whitney v. *California*, 201
Winters v. *Miller*, 158

X-rays, 8

Yudashkin, E. G., 79-80, 83, 84, 187,
  188, 198, 206